PROSTATE CANCER: LIVING WITH IT, LIVING WITHOUT IT

Michael Honeycutt Sr.

ISBN: 197417722X
ISBN-13: 9781974177226

DEDICATION

My dad, Ken Honeycutt, is a prostate cancer survivor. His early detection made it possible for both of us to be alive today. All you have done for us is nothing short of wonderful. My brother Brian Honeycutt, is a prostate cancer survivor. Your work experience is beyond any dream one could imagine. The lifelong commitment to Aikido shows your discipline is a credit to you. My brother Daryl Honeycutt, a twenty-four-year career marine. You were away from us for all those years. I am proud of you and glad to have you back home. My son, Michael Honeycutt Jr. You have achieved so much. I am the proudest father ever. Thanks so much for all you have done to keep us proud and happy for you. Molly Honeycutt. You are our daughter. We are always trying to keep up with you and what you do. That's no easy task for us. It's a whirlwind. Keep it up. My wife, Martha. What a wonderful and giving woman. Your guidance is my inspiration. You are so much fun to be around. Thank you.

INTRODUCTION

What can a man do to avoid getting prostate cancer? There are many speculations, and each year more data is acquired. The projected number of deaths from prostate cancer for 2017 is over 26,700. It is projected that more than 160,000 men will be diagnosed.

Four years and one month from my first elevated PSA result, I had a radical prostatectomy. During those four years, the fear of having prostate cancer was ever present. This is my attempt to help men understand that life goes on even with this concern in their lives.

More importantly I hope that men will be outwardly concerned with this disease. We do not like to talk about having cancer. We do not want to think about the possibility of incontinence or erectile dysfunction.

We like to think prostate cancer only happens to old men. If this happens to me, my life is over. Or at least most of us assume our lives will be over.

I felt the same way. How could I consider surgery that had any possibility of leaving me dribbling in my pants? Worst was the possibility of losing my manhood. Who wants to talk about having those problems? At one time, I never considered discussing the fact that I might not "rise to the occasion." With four years to think about it, I decided this was childish.

I want to share with you some events in my life before and after the radical prostatectomy. Talking about prostate cancer is a man's best defense. Education and loved ones are your allies on the subject. Fear of the unknown has more serious consequences.

Life is great for me now. The decisions I made are not recommended for everyone. I feel I made the right decisions for my situation. What you do with your life depends on your decisions. Who else can help you more than yourself? Your doctors, family, and friends are the most logical choices. Be open with them and especially your doctor. If you feel concerned by what your doctor tells you, get another doctor. You will become more educated and comfortable. This makes all the difference in the world. You need all the ammunition you can get to fight this deadly disease.

QUESTIONS I HAD TO ADDRESS

At what point should a decision be made to remove the prostate if cancer is detected from a biopsy? If detected by a biopsy, how slowly does the cancer move within the prostate? How do you decide to have the prostate removed once you discover you have prostate cancer? What is available other than having the prostate removed? If it is cancerous, how quickly does the cancer progress to the point that it will escape the prostate? These are the questions I wanted answered. It would have made my decisions a lot easier.

The perfect time to have the prostate removed is just before the cancer spreads from the prostate. Trying to time this perfectly is like rolling dice. Once cancer is detected, how long can you wait to have it removed and be 100 percent certain it has not spread?

Today there are many options that were not available in 2001. If you have prostate cancer, do not think that what I did is best for you. Get educated, and discuss your options and their consequences. More information is available today than in 2001.

What level of a PSA (prostate-specific antigen) exam is considered a baseline? The standard during my four years was a baseline of 4.0. I now see articles stating a baseline is of no value. I know two people who had a PSA between 2.0 and 2.5, and prostate cancer was detected by the digital rectal exam. Their biopsies proved it.

CHAPTER 1

INFORMATION

There are approximately 140 million men in America. Each of us needs to be aware of prostate cancer. Once you decide to look at this disease, you need to read about my experience. Every person is different. My experience is meant to be a guideline for you. It is not a direct path for you to follow but provides some basic information.

Why do you need to be concerned with prostate cancer? Once prostate cancer is detected in your body, the decisions you make could decide how long you live. Read the bullets below.

- In 2017, the American Cancer Society estimates that 161,360 men will be diagnosed with prostate cancer. They also estimate that 26,730 men will die from prostate cancer.
- Prostate cancer develops into one of the most painful forms of cancer.
- It moves through the body slowly compared to other types of cancer.
- Usually it goes to the bones, causing them to become very brittle.

- Bodily functions begin to collapse, and pain increases within the body.
- Morphine becomes a friend.
- Chemotherapy, radiation, and hormone treatments are recommended. All are very painful, and time is required to recuperate from the treatments.
- All males are at risk for prostate cancer.
- How will you find out if you have this cancer?

You should know the consequences of doing nothing about the early detection of prostate cancer. Once prostate cancer is detected, living a normal life depends on what advice you take and how fast you act on your doctor's suggestions.

The book *The Prostate* by Patrick C. Walsh, MD, and Janet Farrar Worthington references the American Cancer Society's Department of Epidemiology and Statistics, which estimated two hundred thousand new cases of prostate cancer in 1994. They estimated that thirty thousand men in the United States would die of prostate cancer that year. It is the second-leading kind of cancer affecting men, behind skin cancer. Prostate cancer risk increases significantly with age.

The Prostate states that, in the United States, a man is diagnosed with prostate cancer every three minutes. Every fifteen minutes, a man dies from it in the United States.

The American Cancer Society's website reported that, in 2003, 220,900 new cases would emerge and that 28,900 men would die from prostate cancer. The projection for 2017 is 161,360 new cases and 26,730 men to die from prostate cancer.

This drop in new cases and deaths would indicate that earlier detection is reducing the number of deaths.

Another interesting statistic is that less than 10 percent of men with prostate cancer die within five years of diagnosis. Does this indicate that men are doing something about prostate cancer when diagnosed? Does it mean men are having checkups at earlier ages? With the addition of the PSA test, prostate cancer is being detected much earlier than with the digital rectal exam alone.

Having prostate cancer can be a scary thought. If you have any concerns about what will happen in your life should you be at risk for prostate cancer, read on.

CHAPTER 2

SCREENING

Several screening tests can show the potential risk of prostate cancer. They are not perfect but are easy and can indicate when the prostate is not as it should be. The most common is the digital rectal exam. The doctor inserts his finger up the anus and feels the prostate. The doctor feels for smoothness, size, and hardness. Experience allows the doctor to recognize if something is wrong. That's right: bend over, grab your ankles or knees, and hope it does not take very much time.

According to the National Cancer Institute, web site: www.cancer.gov:

PSA (prostate-specific antigen) is secreted by certain cells of the prostate gland. PSA is a protein produced by the prostate. It liquefies semen and allows sperm to swim freely. A PSA test measures the level of this protein in the blood.

The PSA blood test has a baseline of 4.0. A good result is anything below 4.0. A number above the baseline can be an indication of possible cancer in the prostate.

Many things can affect a PSA result. Most urologists will do several PSA tests over time before deciding if a biopsy is required.

The digital rectal exam can detect prostate cancer even when PSA numbers are low. Inversely, the PSA can yield a high number while the prostate feels fine to the doctor.

My PSA results for this period are below. All the digital rectal exams were fine.

DATE	RESULTS
May 6, 1997	8.0
June 6, 1997	3.3
April 13, 1999	3.5
March 16, 2000	5.4
April 17, 2000	5.0
April 20, 2000	4.0
January 22, 2001	5.3
January 31, 2001	4.5
June 15, 2001	4.2

They were above and below the baseline. At one time, my urologists suggested I may have a higher baseline than the standard 4.0.

A biopsy is next, should either the digital rectal exam or PSA test find evidence that cancer exists. The biopsy is usually performed after several of the other tests or combinations of tests indicate the possibility of cancer.

The samples of the prostate taken during a biopsy are sent to a pathologist for evaluation. A microscopic appearance of prostate cancer cells is called the Gleason Grading System. This might be the most important part of discussions with your urologists. What is the grade?

In the book, *Dear God, It's Cancer* by William S. Fintel, MD, and Gerald R. McDermott, PhD, Publisher: Thomas Nelson, August 7, 1997.

Prostate tumors are graded according to their relative aggressiveness as seen under the microscope by a trained pathologist. Assessing the aggressiveness or "angriness" of the tumor helps determine both treatment and prognosis. The grading system most often used is the Gleason's scale, developed by the V.A. Research Group years ago. The Gleason's score ranges from two to ten, with two being the least angry and ten the most. A linear relationship exists between the Gleason's number and the chance of spread outside the gland. Gleason's scores of two to four have a minimal risk of spread; only twenty-five percent of them move outside the gland. Gleason's scores of eight to ten, on the other hand, have a seventy-five percent chance of spreading beyond the prostate gland.

My Gleason scores from the biopsy were $3 + 3 = 6$. After the surgery, the prostate was examined again. I had the same $3 + 3 = 6$ result.

CHAPTER 3
FIRST AWARENESS

It was a Sunday afternoon after playing golf. My brother Brian asked, "Have you talked to our parents lately?"

"Not since last week. Anything going on?"

"Ken has been diagnosed with prostate cancer," he said. Brian and I always call our father Ken.

"What does that mean? How advanced is the cancer?" I asked.

"I don't know anything about it. They just said he is going for more tests and will know something more definite soon," Brian said.

This was the first time cancer has ever been mentioned for either of my parents. I became fearful my dad had cancer. Cancer seems the most fearsome of all words. Sometimes I feel like the word death is not as scary as cancer. Heart attacks used to be scarier than cancer. Not now. Cancer, to a lot people, means a slow death—a gradual physical worsening. Body parts are removed, and chemotherapy treatments are terrible. Cancer means a painful process toward dying. It's in remission—great news. It's back—sad news. What a roller coaster.

The more I learned about cancer of any type, the more I realized it does not have to be this way. Research has done miracles to increase the life expectancy of people diagnosed with cancer. Early diagnosis has been a leading factor in lengthening our lifespan. Education about the early signs of cancer has probably been the leading reason for our extended life expectancy.

When my dad was admitted to the hospital, I did not understand much about prostate cancer. I knew the prostate could be removed without resulting in many profound consequences. If caught in time, my father would be fine and would live a normal life. The desire is for the cancer to be confined to the prostate. Removing the prostate at this stage would remove 100 percent of the cancer cells.

Dad's surgery was scheduled for the afternoon. While we were saying our goodbyes as he was just about ready to go to surgery, he abruptly said, "I hope I crap all over them during the operation."

We knew he was nervous. We were shocked to hear him say that.

The surgery went well. His expected time in the hospital was three days. The next morning I was in his room. His urologist came by while making his rounds. He was young looking and very confidant. He was drinking a cup of coffee. So this is the famous Dr. Uro my dad is always talking about.

As we were introduced, I immediately liked him. He spoke with concern to my father and mother and was very positive about my dad's surgery. *The next time I need a urologist,* I thought, *he will be my choice.*

Two days later Dad was scheduled to go home. I was at work, which is ten minutes from the hospital. When he was to be released, the plan was for my mother to call when it was time to go over to help her bring him home.

I got a call from mom. Her voice sounded fearful. She said, "Get over here! Ken has passed out, and they have him in intensive care."

"What happened?"

"He was getting up, and he passed out and fell on the floor. I ran and got the nurse. They took him downstairs. Come to the intensive care unit on the first floor. Hurry up!"

Just as I arrived in the ICU waiting room, Dr. Uro walked in with another doctor. They came out of the ICU and asked mom to sit down. The three of them sat on a couch with Dr. Uro in the middle. I sat in a chair facing them.

The other doctor introduced himself. He said he was the hematologist. "Mrs. Honeycutt," he said, "Mr. Honeycutt's blood is not clotting. He has internal bleeding. Whatever went wrong was my fault and had nothing to do with Dr. Uro or your husband's surgery. All the preliminary tests we ran showed that your husband's blood would be able to clot. As you know, he has been on blood thinner for several years due to his frequency of blood clots from his ankle.

"Again, the tests showed that your husband's blood was OK to have this surgery. I am sorry about this and will do everything to make sure he will be fine. Please understand this is my fault and has nothing to do with Dr. Uro. We are going to make some changes in his medication. I will be glad to explain all of this in detail if you like. Simply put, we are going to do what we can to get his blood to clot. I am very sorry about this, and our staff will do everything to get this corrected. He may be in the ICU for several days.

"If there is anything I can do for you or your family, please ask. Just leave a message with any of the nurses in the ICU or call my office. I am very sorry about this."

My father is going to die from internal bleeding, I thought. This doctor was nervous, and he was sincere about my dad being in serious condition.

Dr. Uro's face spoke louder than any words he could have said. He looked mad. He was upset this problem had occurred. I knew he was not happy about a missed diagnosis. He kept moving his head and crossing his legs. He stayed back against the couch and never attempted to say anything.

Dr. Uro waited until the hematologist left the room. He turned to my mom and apologized. "Mr. Honeycutt is not suffering, but he is in a critical state. I will be monitoring him carefully. My office is five minutes from here. I will make sure everything possible is done to correct this."

He never put the blame on anyone. He told us what was going to happen. He said, "Mr. Honeycutt will have swelling, but you should not be concerned. The main thing is we must get the blood to clot. Once that happens Mr. Honeycutt will recover and be as good as new."

Dr. Uro gave us a much better feeling. He kept things simple. He assured us of his help and informed us this would take time. Whatever we needed, he would get for us.

He took us back to see my dad. I do not remember when Brian arrived during this meeting. I was only thinking about how some screw up might have my dad dying of internal bleeding instead of cancer.

He was unconscious but looked good. There were no signs of any problem. He looked comfortable and had normal skin coloring.

Dr. Uro escorted us out into the waiting room. He told us what the hours were for visiting ICU patients. If we wanted to visit at different hours, he would see if that could be possible. He said that rest and allowing the nurses to do their job without visitors was important. If anything should happen, his staff would contact us immediately.

He also said that the other doctor would be monitoring my dad as well and would do everything possible. He finally spoke about the other doctor being the best in Spartanburg at his specialty. He said there are times when tests are not always accurate.

Numbness was upon us after Dr. Uro left. We didn't know what to say to one another. Finally, we talked about what type of arrangements mom wanted to make. Did she want to stay or to be driven home? Frankly, I don't remember what we did or made plans to do. Everything was a blur. Mom would be OK to drive the thirty-minute trip home under normal conditions, but this was not a day for her to drive.

CHAPTER 4

RECOVERING

For several days, dad remained unconscious. His face began to swell some. His scrotal sack was as large as a football. On one visit, Dr. Uro told me he was not worried about the swelling. The only concern was for the blood to start clotting.

Finally, one day he awoke and began to get better. During his recovery time, he was sedated. One day he started talking about a sock hanging on top of the door. I got mad. How can this be happening? He was not in his right mind. My father is the most competent one in our family. He now spoke as if he were completely normal—aside from trying to explain about a sock on top of the door of his room.

He spent eleven days in the ICU and recovered very well. We all were exhausted by the time he was ready to be released. We were there for every visit—four visits a day for fifteen minutes. Some days, as he was getting better, I would arrive early and ring the nurses' station. A nurse would come out and allow me to come in and sit at the foot of his bed and talk. At times we could stay longer than fifteen minutes, provided there were no more than two of us and we were quiet.

When he was released, he was in good physical condition but still had to recover from the surgery. He did very well with his recovery. Mom could take care of him.

Shortly after his surgery, he went for radiation treatments. They were done on an outpatient basis, which was easy for him to take. Dad said they did the radiation in the immediate area where the prostate was located. Dr. Uro wanted to make sure there were no cancer cells left in that area. If the pathology report shows cancer located near the outer surface of the prostate, radiation therapy is recommended as a precaution.

CHAPTER 5
KIDNEY STONES

While doing some paperwork in my office, I felt this terrible pain. It felt like a sharp object piercing me in the lower back.

Where did this come from? Whoa! This is horrible. It will pass, hopefully as quickly as it arrived, I thought. Not so.

Trying to see my family doctor was no good. The receptionist said I could come but would have to be worked in, between appointments. Since the pain was getting worse, I decided instead to go to the emergency room at Mary Black Hospital. It was less than four miles away.

When I arrived at Mary Black hospital, I walked around the parking lot, hoping the pain would go away. It did not. The pain stayed in my lower back, and it was getting worse. I have had some pulled muscles in that area before. They were not as low down in the back, though. Nor were they the same type of pain.

In the emergency room, I talked with the woman at the window for registration. She asked me to go over to another woman at a desk in a corner and fill out the proper paperwork. Once that was finished, I was to return to the window with the paperwork.

I sat down with a woman who was a volunteer. She asked me all the questions about insurance—addresses, phone numbers, which doctors I visited. She finally said, "Explain the problem you have."

I explained my pain and where it was.

She looked at me and said, "Oh, you have a kidney stone."

She led me into the emergency waiting area immediately. With the statement of her diagnosis, I really was at a loss for answers. First, this woman was no nurse or doctor. Was she just guessing? She sounded confident. What is a kidney stone? How did I get one? They are as painful as others have stated. What am I going to have done to me? I wondered. I knew they were not going to give me two aspirin and send me home.

The emergency room was sectioned off with curtains separating the beds. Several people were moving and working on both sides of the room. My section number was three. I could hear a man groaning with pain in section one. He sounded older than me, and from his comments, it sounded like he was feeling awful.

I put on a hospital gown. A cloth draped around the front with the rear end not meeting and a hole for each arm. My butt, back, and legs were all bare to the world. How do people who work in hospitals ever get used to seeing patients in that outfit?

A doctor came up to me and said they wanted to do an x-ray. I was rolled on the gurney into the x-ray area. As I was rolled down a hallway, we passed a young boy of about five years old with his mother. The boy said, "Look, Mama—that man is dead!"

I am very light skinned. Wrapped in a white sheet, with a couple of people dressed in white rolling me down a hall, I guess I looked dead.

Quickly I turned my head to the little boy and said, "Boo."

It scared him, and his mom said, "That's not very nice."

After we turned a corner in the hall, the orderly pushing me started laughing. "You made my day," he said, smiling.

After examining the initial x-ray, the doctor confirmed it was a kidney stone. He wanted to put some liquid in me and do more x-rays. That way he could have a better view to see the size of the stone or if there was more than one. The second x-ray confirmed it was a single big kidney stone.

It was recommended for me to see my urologist with this information. They called my urologist's office to plan for me to visit immediately. Fortunately, his office was just a couple of blocks away. I drove there and met with him.

He said, "The kidney stone needs to be crushed; it is too large to pass. Several years ago, a stone this large was surgically removed. You are very lucky crushing is now an option. The old surgery method required the patient to be cut about halfway around the entire waist. The healing process was terrible. Most people with this surgery had a limp for the rest of their lives."

He called the hospital.

"We are in luck; a mobile unit comes to Spartanburg once a week. They are scheduled to be in Spartanburg tomorrow, and time is available. This is better than the one at the hospital because you are not put to sleep."

The next morning my wife Martha and I were there for the lithotripsy. After the paperwork, I put on the cloth drape again. I sat in a wheelchair and was rolled outside down a ramp into this long Winnebago-type mobile unit. A couple of young people were there and gave me my instructions. They informed me of the procedure and said my urologist should be here soon. Within five minutes Dr. Uro arrived.

I was placed on a flat, hard table. All the equipment was roughly positioned over and under me. Dr. Uro injected me with a steady flow of morphine. A moveable x-ray-looking device was placed over me. I had to move around to get in the correct position. Once I was in position, and the device was set correctly, the procedure started. As I lay relaxed, I felt this pinging going on in my lower-back area.

It continued constantly every few seconds. This went on for about thirty minutes. I imagined a small person under the table hitting me with a dipstick.

Dr. Uro came back to speak with me a couple of times and to make sure I was doing all right. We tried to make small talk. I was really feeling good but wasn't in a silly state of mind.

Finally, Dr. Uro came back and said it was over, and the stone was crushed. All the equipment was removed, and I sat down in the wheelchair. I was given a T-shirt stating that I had been lithotripsied.

Dr. Uro told me to go home and rest. An orderly rolled me away in a wheelchair. Tomorrow I would be able to return to work.

That evening, I developed chills and fever. I stayed in bed for three days with this problem. Yeah, right—go back to work the next day.

About six months later, I had a second kidney stone crushed in the same manner. After passing this crushed stone, I returned to Dr. Uro's office with my second crushed stone. This was three days after the lithotripsy.

While I was there, they drew blood for a PSA test. The results came back three days later with an elevated number of 8.0. Dr. Uro called my home and left a message stating that my PSA was up to 8.0. He felt it had something to do with the stone I passed and wanted to do another PSA test in a month.

CHAPTER 6

REPEAT PSA AND WAIT ON RESULTS

Amonth later I went back to have another PSA test. The visit included another digital rectal examination. This was not my first, but it was my first involving both a PSA and digital rectal exam. This was the beginning of a long combination of PSA tests and digital rectal exams. The cycle of changes from test to test with varying results was a constant mind-control game.

The next day I was on a flight to Leon, France. All during my trip in France, I was worried about the test. I could not get the results for three days.

During the long flight from Atlanta, Georgia, to Leon, France, I stood at the back of the plane just to get out of my seat. A woman was doing the same. During our conversation, she stated that her son-in-law was doing his residency to become a doctor. She told me he was considering urology. I explained about my elevated PSA and then having to retest. She proudly announced that I needed to talk with her husband. He had three biopsies because of elevated PSA results, and all the biopsies came back negative. She retrieved her husband.

We introduced ourselves, and her husband asked about my blood test. I told him about my elevated PSA. The husband told me his history with elevated PSA tests. Three times he had biopsies because of elevated PSA numbers. All three biopsies came back negative.

I asked him to explain the biopsy procedure.

"It was simple," the husband said. "They gave me a shot to relax me but nothing strong. They go up your rectum to get the samples. It takes all of thirty minutes. There is no pain. They barely sedated me. I drove back to work after the last two."

He assured me I had nothing to worry about unless my numbers really jumped, like from a three to a thirteen. I appreciated his encouragement, but I did not believe I would have his history. Nor did I believe his entire story. It sounded to me like more bragging that reality.

We landed in Leon, France, and took a taxi to my hotel located in the middle of the city. The lobby was small with some seats around the immediate area. There was one elevator and a stairway, and to the left of the lobby was a bar. My room was typical of the rooms I have stayed in during my previous trips to Europe. It was small and simple with black and white colors and wood furnishings.

I rested for a couple of hours. Forcing myself not to sleep, to get my body acclimated to the current time zone, was always a problem. I did get up, though, and got dressed and took a walk around the city.

There was a huge water display in an area close to my hotel. The water display had a walking area around its perimeter, which was about thirty feet. Next to half the walking perimeter was a three-lane street. On the other half was a huge sidewalk leading through several stores. It was Sunday, and people were walking around enjoying the day. It was interesting to watch people on this lazy day. I knew tomorrow this area would be filled with people and automobiles rushing to their destinations, but today was a day of relaxation.

After my walk, I returned to the hotel and went to the bar. The bar was to the left of the registration desk in the same area that was used for continental breakfast. I nodded to the bartender and said hello; he returned my hello.

"What is your favorite local beer," I asked.

"Yes, I get," he replied. He opened a door behind him and took out a Budweiser.

"Glass?" he asked.

"Yes."

He brought a bowl of nuts and set them down in front of me.

He did not speak very much English. He assumed I wanted an American beer. I prefer local beer in Europe, but I didn't want to have much of a discussion with anyone. I was tired. I planned to drink a couple beers and go to sleep early.

The beer nuts were good, and the beer was, strangely enough, rather cold. Beer in Europe is kept at room temperature or barely chilled. I decided to stick with Budweiser; it was probably the coldest because no one ever drank it.

I began to wake up and feel better. The bartender looked after me, keeping me full of nuts and asking if I was ready for another beer when my bottle got low. The bartenders in Europe seemed to watch their customers closely and make sure they were served promptly.

"Is there an excellent restaurant nearby?" I asked.

"Yes." He gave me a small card for a restaurant. "Ten minutes," he said, pointing to his right.

I walked to the restaurant and had a very satisfying meal. They spoke English. Since it was Sunday and very early, I was the first customer.

The next morning I met my escort. The initial contact was a fellow American. He has a business connecting American companies with French companies or vice versa. He had prepared the trip, and the meeting I was to have with the owner of a French company. We planned to discuss the possibility of licensing his technology and marketing it in North America. We were to spend a couple of days together so I could see the company and visit some of his customers.

Once we finished the introductions, we drove to the company headquarters. The streets were heavy with traffic. People were rushing around. As we drove by the water fountain I visited yesterday, it bore little resemblance to what I saw the day before. People were hurrying around, and there was very little time for relaxation.

The office belonged to a technical company that did software writing and housed hardware.

It was a small company like mine. Secretarial and accounting comprised the rest of the office. I did enjoy seeing Oracle manuals in the offices. I owned stock in Oracle.

Driving through France in a two-door BMW 3 Series on the interstate and mountain roads was quite an experience. The speed was much faster than in America. We drove into a large city and then through some small towns. In the small towns, the doors of businesses and homes opened onto the sidewalk, which connected to the road. Everything was close together. There were no yards—just the road, a small sidewalk, and the buildings. If we were to go off the road, we would be in someone's bedroom before we had a chance to get back onto the road. The countryside and small villages were very attractive and enjoyable to see. All the villages seemed to be closed; I saw very few people.

We ate in a couple of small villages that provided excellent food and service. One evening we went to a huge shopping area in Leon. We walked around cobbled streets and looked in shops. The restaurant was small with a cobbled floor and brick walls. Our food was delivered to the table. It was delicious, and there was so much. I somehow managed to eat it all to avoid disappointing my escort or the chef.

One afternoon we got in a discussion about hobbies. The owner of the French company said he rode horses cross-country. They would ride up to twenty miles on a cross-country trip. The first time we stopped the car after this discussion, he opened the trunk of his car to show me some of his riding equipment. He had a bridle and a small saddle—not like western saddles—and a black hard hat. I also noticed about eight two-liter bottles of water. I asked him about the water. He said that he drank two of those bottles a day.

Unfortunately, my thoughts were not about this beautiful countryside. What will I do if I have prostate cancer? I was depressed. I hated hospitals and wanted to avoid them and any type of surgery.

The last night before flying home, I spoke to Martha on the telephone. She said the doctor called and said my PSA was normal. I was very relieved.

CHAPTER 7

BREAST CANCER

Shortly after returning from Leon, I went to dinner with Bill, a close friend all my life. His wife Deana had just passed away after fighting breast cancer for three years.

"Deana worked and saved for retirement. She never made it to retirement. I will not worry anymore about saving for retirement. You never know when you will be gone," Bill said.

This was true. I was saving all this money for retirement. Why? Within a week, I bought a BMW.

Deana's passing and my worries about prostate cancer gave me a different perspective on life. You never know what will happen to you. You cannot expect to live forever, but you want to be able to live a long and healthy life. Now I realized this was not always true. I would try to live in the present and save some money for the future even though I may not be around for that future.

Bill met Deana when she was a student at Limestone College in our hometown of Gaffney, South Carolina. They got married shortly after Bill served on active duty in the US Navy. I went to a couple of small parties at their home when I was home on leave from the navy.

Before moving back to Gaffney, they lived in Chester, South Carolina. Bill was a highway patrolman and had a locksmith's shop. Parts of the movie *Chiefs* were filmed in Chester during their stay. Bill was lifting weights big time. He played the part of the strongman in a carnival in the movie. I had to laugh at the picture of him in an animal-print loin cloth. It went down to his knees, and he was standing there holding a barbell loaded with weights.

Those three years were a roller coaster for Deana, Bill, and their children, Jason and Brooke. There were bad results from tests and then satisfactory results. They would announce that her cancer was in remission, and the next report would show another occurrence of cancer.

She went through chemotherapy treatment three times. After the chemo, she could not be exposed to anyone for fear of catching something her body could not fight off, so she stayed inside. As she got better, we would visit. Even then she told the greatest stories.

They searched for ways of healing or getting the cancer into remission everywhere and anywhere. Deana wanted to try some natural healing. They found all they wanted and more. There were all types of money-making schemes promoting cures. I believe they briefly tried one and quickly realized there was a small economy preying on cancer victims. It reminded me of traveling-medicine shows in the Wild West.

They contacted the John Wayne Cancer Institute. I went with Bill to FedEx all her medical records there. She and Bill hoped this would be a good chance for her; they were willing to try anything. The John Wayne Cancer Institute turned her down. Her cancer was too advanced. This really hurt them emotionally. It was probably the final factor that led them to believe there would be no cure or possibility of getting the cancer in remission.

Deana was in good enough health to participate in Brooke's wedding. It was a wonderful feeling for all of us to know she was physically able to play an active part in this wedding.

One day I saw Deana eating lunch at a restaurant with some of the other teachers from the school where she works. She was telling some story and everyone was laughing. We talked for a few minutes. She indicated she was eating a large lunch because there was no need for her to diet anymore. She was going to eat what she wanted. She knew that soon she would have no appetite.

During her last days, Deana was hospitalized. I went to visit the family one evening at the hospital. When I got there, she was still in the room and had just passed away. A sheet was put over her except for her left foot. The emotions in the room were those of sadness and relief. Bill's aunt and uncle, Dean and Tootsie, were there along with all Deana's family.

As I walked from the room, headed out to my car, Big O was just coming in to visit. I told Big O the news. We got in his car and drove to Bill's home. He called his girlfriend Judy, and I called Martha to tell her the news. At Bill's home, people started coming in. We sat and had small talk. Bill arrived, and I could see he was glad to have some people around; it was apparent he did not want to be alone.

Deana's funeral was tough for all of us. Her family did well. I know they were exhausted and glad to know her pain was over and that she had gone on to a better place.

At the end of the church service, Martha and I were in the car waiting on the procession to the cemetery. The church bell rang a single chime every fifteen seconds. It kept ringing, and I broke down and cried. "I wish they would stop ringing that damn bell", I said.

CHAPTER 8

APRIL 13, 1999 | PSA 3.5

Gaffney, South Carolina, is my home. The long-established Shuford-Hatcher Funeral Home was a family-owned business. They were in the process of selling to a large company with many locations across the United States.

Before Shuford-Hatcher sold, they had a sale on crypts and grave sites. Dad bought two, for my mother and him.

A few years later, as my mother was getting worse with her cirrhosis of the liver, she began to worry about dying and was concerned about the location of the crypts, which were outdoors.

After much discussion, Dad agreed to trade their two outside crypts for two inside ones. The new owners had taken over, and they refused to exchange the existing crypts for two inside without a significant price increase.

I called Brian and said, "We should buy the two from Dad."

"What will we do with them?"

"We can sell them," I said. "If not, we can be buried in them."

"Wouldn't you want to be buried beside me?" I asked. "Or the first one in the family to die gets them and pays the other one for the remaining one. Then you will be beside Maurine or vice versa."

"OK, if you think we can sell them," he said.

We bought the two crypts, and Dad bought two more inside.

A month or so after our mother died, Martha, Dad, and I visited my mother's crypt. Dad said he called his neighbors, the Johnsons, to come look at the two crypts Brian and I owned. The Johnsons were interested in buying them. Martha and I left, and Dad waited on the Johnsons to arrive.

Now that the new owners had taken over the funeral home, an inexperienced staff was hired. Dad called me the next day, sounding very upset. "The Johnsons," he said. "I took them to see where the two crypts were located. There was a body already buried in one of your crypts! This morning I went to the funeral home office and threatened to sue them."

"What is the problem, Mr. Honeycutt?" the woman had asked my dad.

"There is somebody buried in my son's crypt."

The woman pulled out a layout of the crypts and got the identification numbers. After looking up the owner, she said we owned them. Upon looking further, she found that another family had bought the same ones. A mistake had been made, and it was their fault. Another family purchased the crypts just after dad bought them.

"We will move the casket immediately," she said.

"I am not going to have my sons buried where someone else was buried," he said. "We want our money back now, or I will own this place."

"I need to talk with my supervisor who is out of town," she said. "Tomorrow I will have an answer for you, Mr. Honeycutt."

Naturally the call never came. Dad called me and said to get a lawyer. I wanted to avoid any confrontation that required a lawyer, so I called the woman and listened to her story. They accidentally sold the crypts twice. With the change in ownership of the cemetery, this was completely overlooked. She apologized.

"What can be done?" I asked.

"I called my boss, and he told me to have you select two more at another location but in the same price range."

"We will consider taking two others at another location." I said. "Have your supervisor call me. If I don't hear from him by tomorrow, we must contact a lawyer." She agreed to tell him.

That afternoon her supervisor called me at work. He apologized and said they made a mistake. "Your crypts were sold so close together that your purchase had not been recorded before being sold again," he said.

"I need something to feel that you are willing to pay for your mistake," I said. "I do not want very much but something to show that you really are sorry for the mistake you made."

"What do you want?" he asked.

"Our choice of the remaining crypts and a free bronze inscription."

"OK, that is fair," he agreed.

Dad contacted The Johnsons. They chose another location and purchased the crypts. That left Brian and me out in the cold.

A few hundred yards behind the crypts, I noticed a small ditch. Maybe when we die I can get someone to pitch our bodies in this ditch and cover us with lime, put some dirt over us, stack some rocks over the dirt, and put a wooden cross in the rocks. A wooden inscription could say something like, "Here lie the Honeycutt boys, so stingy they sold their own burial plots."

CHAPTER 9

MARCH 16, 2000 | RESULT 5.4

Oh hell! I have prostate cancer. Wild thoughts and many questions needed to be addressed. Am I going to need surgery? Do I go through with an operation? Do I do seed implants or radiation? Will I become impotent? Am I going to piss in my pants the rest of my life? Has the cancer spread to other parts of my body? What caused this? Too much or too little sex in my life? Did my vasectomy have anything to do with it? Did I break a chain letter? What happens next?

Prior to this result, my life was mentally on a high. I was self-sufficient and of the feeling that I could do no wrong. I could overcome most anything.

All that changed after the reading of 5.4 on my PSA results. I had cancer, and I needed help.

A new reality was settling in my thoughts. Getting advice and knowledge, improving my physical and mental state, and getting closer to God became priorities.

Fear is an important theme of the Bible. There are many references to people fearing God. It is a wake-up call to something that has happened in the stories. The way of overcoming fear is to have faith in God. As your faith increases, fear is reduced or goes away.

Eventually I changed my thoughts, realizing I was not in complete control. God had a plan for me, and I needed to find it. There was something more important than material things. By partnering with God, I could overcome fear of the unknown.

Could I go through chemotherapy? I saw a Deana go through chemo. I knew that I would and was sure Martha and Dr. Uro would talk me into doing chemo if required. But how I would hate to go through it.

Radiation and hormone treatment—I think these are as bad as chemo. I saw a person go through these treatments. It was hard on him. Radiation burned the crap out of him in certain areas. The hormone treatments were bad as well. He said that when that hormone injection came into his body, he wanted to find a hiding place and scream.

Beyond the treatments, what about life?

What if I died? What happens? All my worries would be over. No more worrying about prostate cancer. No more worries about life itself. No financial worries—nothing. It would be over as far as living on this earth as a human.

No, it is not over. When someone dies, there are people left to carry on without them. Martha and Michael would continue with their lives without me.

Friends would miss me but nothing like my immediate family. Friends would continue with their lives while remembering me.

Martha and Michael would have to make serious decisions that I usually make. Their lives would change, but both were strong and would adapt.

This also meant a change in my relationship with God. Where could I go to find out what I needed to comfort me as my life continued? I needed to find or get a miracle. How is a miracle obtained? I doubted that I would get touched by God and that the prostate cancer would just go away and I would be instantly healed.

There is another form of healing that is possible. That is the healing of gradually getting better. It can be in the form of medicine, surgery, and asking God for healing. God will give me an out to become whole again, I thought. He always does. It is our responsibility to find it. Prayer is a start.

My praying became more serious. I believed more that God does help those who get serious about their faith. I became a wiser person in my faith in God and Jesus Christ. I was probably fooling myself about my faith until this happened. It wasn't until my diagnosis that it became clear to me that I need to become wiser in my faith.

Praying, reading the Bible, and got more involved with my church. This took me to a higher level in my life. I became more alert to my surroundings and the people around me. I didn't want to miss something Jesus might be trying to tell me. I must be alert to his teaching.

Could having prostate cancer be a test from God for me? Did he challenge me with the ordeal of having prostate cancer? Was it a test of my endurance? Was it a test of my faith?

One thing that was for sure was God knew the outcome, and I did not. My thoughts were that the cancer resulted from evolution; heredity; or the invasion of my body through food, the air, or the environment—Agent Orange in Vietnam, the mosquito spray we followed on our bicycles as children, or some toxins that were sprayed onto our food. Who knows?

My prostate cancer was discovered early because of God, my urologist's knowledge, Martha, and my perseverance. God, knowing the outcome, wanted it to be discovered in the initial stages. I could listen to people and receive God's desire. The reasons for my early detection surely relates to the old saying "God isn't finished with me yet."

During one of my earliest visits to Dr. Uro for kidney stones, he told me the possibility of that I would have prostate cancer was 50 percent higher than normal because my father had had it. He said it could be heredity.

Age, family history, and diet are some things specialists feel can affect someone's chance of getting prostate cancer. The environment and occupations are other considerations, but there is uncertainty around those two areas.

Hardly any Japanese men die from prostate cancer, yet Japanese, American, and all men throughout the world have the same probability of having prostate cancer as shown in autopsies. These were autopsies performed on men regardless of the cause of death. Some autopsies attempt to explain why so many deaths of American men result from the environment. Some studies have shown that when men change their environment, they assume the cancer risk associated with the country in which they live.

As always, the implication is that our high-fat Western diet contributes to the problem. For this reason, a significant number of articles recommend that Americans drink green tea and soy milk. Of course, Americans need to reduce the high-fat foods that we all love and enjoy. Obviously, the best thing to do is to move to Japan.

The topic of prostate cancer running in the family is of great interest to me. There seems to be a close association between family history and a man's risk of developing prostate cancer. Johns Hopkins shows a link between family history and a man's probability of developing prostate cancer. A man's risk of developing prostate cancer is 13 percent. If your father or brother had it, your risk is 26 percent. Add another brother and your risks increases. There is another statistic: if you have a father or brother who had been diagnosed with prostate cancer, it is more likely to strike you at a younger age. If you have a family member diagnosed with prostate cancer, I recommend you begin examinations at the age of forty.

Dad was diagnosed with prostate cancer at the age of sixty-one; I was diagnosed at age fifty-three. Family history gave me an early-warning signal. If someone in your family is diagnosed with prostate cancer, what are your immediate thoughts? For me, I wondered do I or will I have it? I became more interested in my personal condition concerning the potential of being affected by prostate cancer.

Dr. Uro and I discussed all the available options for treating prostate cancer. He told me that it moves very slowly and that I did not have to make a quick decision. He stated that my numbers were low. That was a good sign. Another good sign was that my numbers were gradually rising; they had not jumped to a high number.

"We need to do another rectal exam," he said.

Perhaps he might feel something that would be helpful in the discovery. Apparently, he did, too. Of all the digital rectal exams I've had, this one was the longest and most painful. He prodded, plunged, gouged, and curled his finger in every way imaginable. "It feels normal," he said as he finished. "Perhaps a little enlarged, but that is expected for your age."

Good. I'm glad something feels normal. I sure don't.

I cruised the Internet to learn more about prostate cancer and found a lot of information. Many people had questions that helped me understand a lot of the terms used. Gleason scores kept coming up. The term "Uro" referred to urologists. I found many people asking questions on behalf of a father, husband, or other relative. I think there were more of these people asking questions than those of us who were possible candidates for having prostate cancer. Maybe some of the people were the affected person but didn't want anyone to know. I think most of the people were asking for people who were not Internet literate, or they just wanted to be of help to someone they cared about.

Some people recommended natural cures. This place in St. Louis kept coming up. The claim was that there was a cure without surgery. Drinking green tea and soy milk and eliminating fried foods were very popular suggestions. Other advice included seeing specialists in natural fields and certain surgeons or radiologists.

I found recommendations for specialists covering all parts of the United States.

I had a brief conversation with a man who lived in San Diego. We chatted a little about having prostate cancer. I remember him commenting that no one told him eating fried foods would increase your risk of prostate cancer. He said he wished he had known this several years earlier. I commented that if I had known fried foods had an effect, it would've made no difference to me. I was always one of those people who thought nothing would happen to me. It was always someone else. After thinking about it, he agreed that he would probably have done nothing about changing his diet either.

The following scenario seemed to reoccur frequently: a urologist will recommend surgery, a nutritionist will recommend changing your habits, and a radiologist will recommend radiation. What was ultimately said over and over was that no specialists in their field really knew the other specialties and would never recommend anything except their special field. Of course, there were comments that they all do it for the money.

Personally, I do not accept these thoughts. I think that a specialist knows his field better than another field. As a result, a specialist makes suggestions from his or her expertise and experience. Specialists also know from experience and knowledge when to suggest that a patient see another specialist in a different field. No urologist is going to treat a patient with radiation or herbs but will instead refer you to a specialist in those fields.

I realized I was on my own and would have to make my decisions myself. That thought always resurfaced. The more I read and heard from these people, it became very clear: you must make your own choices, and there is not enough information to tell you the exact course of action to take.

CHAPTER 10

APRIL 17, 2000 | RESULT 5.0 | UNWELCOME NEWS AGAIN

Dr. Uro wanted me to do this test after last month's reading of 5.4. He was confident my numbers would go down. At the time of the last test, I had been taking Vioxx, an antibiotic. He thought the medication could have affected the PSA result.

When I got the 5.0, I was sort of relieved since it was down 0.4 from a 5.4. Dr. Uro also felt good about this. He suggested my baseline might be higher than 4.0. There are people who have a higher baseline PSA naturally, without having prostate cancer. I hoped this might be my situation.

He was not so excited about the reduction from 5.4 to 5.0, however, that he forgot about the dreaded digital rectal exam.

"I need to check your prostate again," he said.

"It was just thirty days ago that I had one."

"I may have missed something last time. Or there could have been a change in your prostate. You cannot be completely sure since we can't see it," he said.

This one was nothing like the last one. It was more like the routine type. Maybe routine is not a good word to use. But in my case, it was routine.

Next time I must see him, I will be prepared. After the nurse leaves the room and closes the door, I will make my move. Pull down my pants and underwear. As soon as I hear him grab the door, I will turn around and bend over, holding my ankles.

"Hello, Doc! I'm in a hurry—double-parked outside."

CHAPTER 11

APRIL 20, 2000

It was time for a physical with my family internist. We talked about my PSA being around 5.0 from the results of the physical. These results concerned him because it was above the 4.0 baseline. I felt good because I had dropped almost a full point. I discussed the other numbers of previous PSA tests with him. He repeated what Dr. Uro had told me some time ago:

Different laboratories doing the PSA could have different numbers. Both doctors were referring to the possibility that the same blood sample sent to two different labs for evaluation could show different numbers. Having a PSA test can be like having a blood pressure test: it can vary from time to time and from machine to machine.

I suggested that I did not need a digital rectal exam because I'd had several since my last physical. No need to go to that cave.

Dr. Intern did not agree, so down went the pants.

Martha and I decided not to worry about it anymore. I was OK, and I would live to be one hundred. My PSA results were not escalating. If I really had prostate cancer, then my numbers should be closer to 10.0 or going in that direction. I was floating between 4.0 and 5.0, so perhaps my baseline is above 4.0.

CHAPTER 12

SEVERAL PSA TESTS

On January 22, 2001, it was time for another PSA test just to pacify everyone.

Damn it! A 5.3 result! My results are elevated again. What in the world is going on? I was on no medication. I was trying to do everything suggested by everyone. Some suggestions included not eating red meat or fried food, following an Asian diet, and drinking green tea and soy milk. I tried all that briefly except the Asian diet. Green tea was OK. I enjoyed soy milk. It was possible for me to regularly drink these things because of the way they taste.

It was time again for the digital rectal exam. I forgot to do my show-and-tell act.

"Why do they call it digital," I asked.

"Because it's one finger, a single digit," he said.

Thank goodness it's not called a dual rectal exam—or a five-finger rectal exam.

Surely you have heard the most frequently told jokes about the digital rectal exam. The most common is the patient telling the urologist that he does not want to feel two hands on his shoulder while getting a rectal exam.

Dr. Uro wanted me to come back in a week and have another test.

January 31, a week later, I had another PSA at my urologist's office. The result was 4.5 *My PSA is going down*, I thought. *That's good.* But it is not below 4.0. Dr. Uro assured me that if I had prostate cancer, my numbers would be going up and not tracking downward. He said, "Let's try it again in six months."

Now I was sure my baseline was higher than the 4.0 used by everyone in the entire world. No need to be concerned until my PSA gets above 6.0.

"Let me check your prostate," Dr. Uro said.

"I just got a digital rectal exam last week. Can we avoid it this time?"

"Nope. It's a good test, and something may have developed, or I may have missed something," he said.

June 15, 2001, six months later, I had another PSA. The result was 4.2.

If you have been in a urologist's office, you know there are at least two twenty-ounce tubes of K-Y Jelly. One has been opened and is usually half empty. There are others in boxes, perfectly stacked at the back of the desk next to a box of rubber gloves and tissue boxes. Behind one of the cabinet doors, I bet, there is a two-by-four he uses to stick up my butt.

I think urologists use about half of a twenty-ounce tube for each digital rectal exam. When they finish, it requires almost a box of tissues to clean yourself. Cleaning yourself with a tissue, trying to get a half pound of K-Y Jelly off that location, is awkward to say the least. One handful of tissues is not enough.

My results were going down. Wow! That was good, but I still was not out of the woods. Dr. Uro said, "You do not have it. I feel good about the last two tests' numbers declining." After a long discussion, he recommended that I have a biopsy just to make everyone feel good about these last numbers. A biopsy was much more reliable for diagnosing prostate cancer.

He explained the procedure. "We take eight sections of the prostate in the biopsy. If one shows up as cancerous, then you have it. If none show up in the eight sections, there is a very good chance you do not have it. But those eight sections could possibly miss a part that may be cancerous. The eight sections come from separate parts of the prostate. It would be a very good indication if you have it or not."

CHAPTER 13

JUNE 6, 2001 COLONOSCOPY | JUNE 8, 2001 BIOPSY

Martha was scheduled to have a colonoscopy. We arrived at the outpatient location of the hospital for the procedure. An employee of the hospital filled out our paperwork and instructed us to go through a door and wait in the lobby. They would call for Martha. I led Martha through the wrong door into a room with about twenty or so cables used for a colonoscopy hanging on a wall. They were long and black and wide in circumference. They looked like black fire hoses.

I announced to Martha, "Those are the tubes that will be inserted into your rectum!"

"Shut up," she said, turning to leave the room.

Martha was given a patient gown and asked to step into a changing room to put it on. When she returned, she was instructed to lay on a bed until another person came for her. A nurse came over and discussed the procedure. Martha expressed an interest in seeing it on the monitor just like Katie Couric did on television. The nurse laughed and said to tell them in the next room.

They showed her where the monitor was located so she could watch if she wanted, but she was out so fast she didn't see the procedure.

After the procedure, the doctor came out, woke Martha up, and told us the results were good. He said, "There were a couple of polyps the size of a BB. I removed them."

"A BB?" I asked. "That's big, isn't it?"

"No, we see some the size of golf balls," he said.

Martha was very draggy. "I didn't get to see my colonoscopy on the monitor the way Katie Couric did," she said.

After the doctor left, the nurse came back to get Martha out of the bed to get it ready for the next group. Martha complained, "I didn't get to see the colonoscopy like Katie Couric."

"We can have them do it again. You could stay awake and watch," I suggested. The nurse laughed.

"That's OK," she said pathetically. She was not interested in that.

I drove her home and put her to bed. She slept most of the day. When she woke she was fine. Her appetite was back.

I agreed to have my colonoscopy. It was scheduled for June 4, 2001—four days before my biopsy. Once I realized this, I called Dr. Uro's office to ask if it was OK to have both tests so close together.

"I have a prostate biopsy scheduled for June the eighth," I said to a nurse over the phone. "I didn't realize it, but I have a colonoscopy scheduled four days earlier. I am sure you realize where both procedures are performed?"

"Yes, sir, I do," she said.

"Is having both done four days apart going to be a problem?" I asked, laughing.

She laughed and said, "I have never been asked that question. Let me ask one of the doctors about this. Can you hang on a second and let me find a doctor?"

"Sure, but try and keep a straight face when you ask one."

"Oh, here comes Dr. Uro. I'll ask him," she said.

She put her hand over the receiver. I could not hear completely, but I did detect that she was asking in an informal way with a little comical tone in her voice.

I heard Dr. Uro laugh. Her hand must have moved away from the receiver. I also heard him say "I don't think there is anything wrong if the colonoscopy is done before the biopsy."

She spoke into the receiver, "We think this will not be a problem. Just do not do the colonoscopy after the biopsy."

The day of the colonoscopy, I met with Dr. Rambo, the gastrologist. He knew our family and asked about my dad.

"He is doing fine; thanks for asking," I said. "I have a prostate biopsy in four days. My PSA is a little elevated. They want to do a biopsy. I think it's just to satisfy everybody," I said.

"I hope you do well. Prostate cancer is nothing to play around with. I am glad they scheduled you for a biopsy," Dr. Rambo said. "You are doing all the right things by scheduling a colonoscopy at your age. I feel strongly that nobody would have colon cancer if they had a colonoscopy every few years after the age of forty-five. By doing so, cancer can be detected in the initial stages and corrected," Dr. Rambo said.

A nurse gave me an injection during our conversation. While Dr. Rambo was talking, I fell asleep. I woke up feeling drowsy in the recovery room, and Martha helped me get dressed. The results showed some small polyps that were removed. On the way home, I made Martha stop to get me a giant hamburger. I'd never slept so well as I did after I got home that evening.

CHAPTER 14

THE BIOPSY

The biopsy was scheduled for June 8, 2001. I dreaded that day. The results would show one of two things:

1. One of the eight sections has a cancerous cell, proving I have prostate cancer.
2. All eight sections are negative, implying I do not have it. But I still cannot be assured 100 percent that I do not have it. The eight sections taken might have missed any part of the prostate that has cancer cells.

With odds like that, Las Vegas should take the gamble.

The day came for the biopsy. Martha went with me to drive me home. The place was an office in the same building as Dr. Uro's. I recognized some of the nurses as employees of Dr. Uro.

Dr. Uro came out and informed Martha and me what they would be doing. He said, "There will be some minor discomfort but not enough to worry about."

"I feel confident you do not have prostate cancer; your numbers are regressing instead of escalating," he said. "But I do want to be assured and have all of us at ease. This will be a very good indication that you do not have it."

I put on the patient's gown. I was beginning to get accustomed to these gowns. They rolled me to the back of the area. I was given a shot for relaxation and instructed to turn onto my side.

Something was inserted into my rectum. I heard this snap, and it felt like something was pinched inside me. This was done eight times. Every time I heard the snap, I expected the pinch. I tried to stay still and did a respectable job of doing so, but I knew it was coming and mentally tried not to flinch.

CHAPTER 15
THE BIOPSY RESULTS

Dr. Uro's office was to call in a couple of days to schedule a follow-up visit to go over the results. After four days and no call, I called his office. His nurse called the pathology department. They said the results were complete and they would send them to Dr. Uro's office. We scheduled a meeting the next day. When I got to the office, I told a nurse why I was there. She looked through my file and some other places and could not find my results. She called pathology. They were going to fax them immediately. She escorted me to a private room and said the doctor would be in shortly.

I waited quietly in a private patient's room with a thousand thoughts running through my mind. I prayed for this to be negative and to be over. But deep inside, I knew my results were not good.

I heard a noise outside my room. Someone was putting my file in the small box attached to the door. My biopsy results were in that box. I got up and opened the door, grabbed my file, and went back inside.

My hands shook as I opened my file. On top was a faxed copy with a diagram of what looked like an oddly shaped circle. It was supposed to be a prostate. There were eight sections squared within this circle. Three of them had an *X* on them.

There was no need to try to understand the writing, but I read it anyway. All I understood was the diagram explained three of the eight sections came back for positive cancer cells.

After I returned the file to the box on the door, I shut the door and sat down. I was isolated. Here I was, waiting in a room for a doctor to come in and give me the results of whether I have cancer or not. And I know the results. My body was as tough as a five-dollar steak, and I felt as though it had betrayed me. What would I tell Martha? I was glad I had come alone. I wanted to be alone.

Shortly after, I felt relieved. Now I knew. No more bad results causing fear and concern followed by satisfactory results causing joy and back again. All that was over. No more consultations with Dr. Uro trying to explain my unusual PSA swings. The roller coaster ride was over. Now it was time to move on to another carnival ride. Only this one was more life-threatening. I would make the most difficult decision I'd ever made in my life. Which carnival ride would I buy a ticket for?

I heard Dr. Uro's voice in the hall. I heard him grab my file, and the door opened. He entered while looking at my file. He did not have his usual smile and friendly welcome. He was showing concern and complexity. He did not say hello but kept looking over the file.

He sat down close to me and told me, "The results came back with three sections being positive. I am sorry for thinking you did not have prostate cancer."

This was the second time I'd seen him at a loss for words. After regrouping, he was good at explaining things. He's the type who stays with a patient until all questions are answered.

He recomposed himself and began telling me what the pathology report showed. He told me again that he was sorry about the results but that the pathology numbers looked very good.

He informed me that we had exposed the cancer early. All the Gleason numbers indicate it is in its initial stages and should not have spread outside the prostate.

He wanted me to talk with Martha and arrange to come back to discuss the options and anything else we wanted to talk about.

When I walked out of the private room, Dr. Uro was talking, but I do not remember what he was saying. It was some words of encouragement. I was in a daze.

There were two nurses who knew me from all my many visits and discussions about my PSA results. One of them came over and said, "I am sorry, and we will do everything we can for you."

The other nurse came over and said, "I am sorry. I know you're going to beat this. You are in much better health than most of our patients, and they beat this all the time."

After thanking them both, I continued walking. They were being nice. I was not very polite. I was in a daze. I made an appointment at the front office to come back for another visit.

I rarely ever drive without the radio on. This time I turned it off and drove home. Still churning over the last hour in my mind, I decided to tell Martha straight-out when I got home.

I pulled into the garage, got out of my car, and walked into the kitchen. I told Martha the news. She immediately responded to all the positive things. She said, "It has been detected early. You can get it out of your body and continue life as normal. We need to prepare and make sure we do the right thing and have a long and happy life together. God will help us through this. We need to get started on this and get it over with as soon as possible."

CHAPTER 16

WHAT'S NEXT

Of all the things Martha has done for me, the most important was to guide me to positive thoughts and to look to God for answers. She did not show signs of pity. She did not tell me she was sorry; she talked about how everything would be all right. We have gone through other things, and they turned out all right. She never reacted with sorrow. I have always loved this characteristic of hers. I do not show her, but I depend on this from her. I would be lost without her.

The day came for us to visit Dr. Uro. We dressed leisurely. It the afternoon. We were very late in getting to see him after our scheduled appointment time. I pointed out to Martha that this man would take all the time a patient needed when visiting him. Therefore, he is usually late in getting to us. I always schedule my appointments for the early morning.

Martha had her questions written down. She and I discussed our individual questions so we would not be redundant, but most of our questions were the same. Of course, I wanted to save some to discuss with the doctor alone.

When Dr. Uro arrived, we did not go into a patient's room. He escorted us to a more relaxed room with soft chairs and nice furniture. We asked all the questions one would expect to ask.

"How dangerous is the surgery?" she asked.

"No more than any other surgery."

"What would be the recovery time?" she asked.

"Two weeks with a catheter," he said. "This is to allow the urethral track to heal and not close. After the removal of the tube, it'll be four or five weeks before returning to work."

Incontinence would require me to wear a diaper for a brief period. Then something like a feminine napkin was recommended. After that I would be normal and could forget that part except for occasional leaks. He informed me these leaks occur in men and women even without this type of surgery. If he could come up with a cure for incontinence, he would be very wealthy. I had better than a 95 percent chance of recovering from incontinence.

Impotence had less a percentage of recovery than incontinence.

"About fifty percent of our patients seem to recover from impotence over time," he said. "Dr. Walsh states that eighty percent of his patients recover, but I doubt that number," he said.

"At your age and with the early detection, you should have a better than fifty percent of recovering from impotence," he said. "All people are different. I had one patient who claimed to have an erection the day after surgery in the hospital with the catheter in him."

I laughed at that comment. It had to hurt with a catheter.

"There are ways to get around impotence. There is Viagra and using injections. These injections would be in the penis. An erection would occur, guaranteed, and last for a long time. I had a patient and friend who used it and thought it was great. He said he wished he had been introduced to it earlier."

Dr. Uro had prescribed Viagra before when I was having a problem. I went to him because Martha felt it was in my mind. I never told her I used Viagra, which did work.

I was afraid he was going to mention that he had prescribed Viagra to me before in front of Martha. I was sweating bullets, but he did not mention it.

"You probably should use the injection first," he said.

As he talked, all I could think about was sticking a needle in my penis. My legs closed and my knees shivered. Who was going to do this for me? Me? I doubted it. There would be no sex because I would pass out. Martha hates needles, so I know she wouldn't do it.

Maybe I could do it if I did it quickly. Use it as though it were a dart. Throw it in the penis. Squeeze the serum out and give a quick jerk to pull it out. This would have me dancing around the room, and not in a Pee-wee Herman way.

I would be standing there, naked, with a syringe in my left hand, and Martha in bed waiting to make love, watching me with a look of curiosity. I would stretch my penis and pitch the syringe into this little noodle. Pain would shoot up to my brain. I would dance around the room, jumping and saying, "Oh God! Oh God!" After settling down, I would look at the needle hanging onto my penis, inject the serum, give a big jerk, and out it would come. My penis would get hard enough to drill.

To hell with a needle, I thought. *I am not going that route.*

Dr. Uro brought me back to reality. "The injection will not hurt. It would be inserted where there are few nerves. You can put on some Frank Sinatra music, and in about ten to fifteen minutes, you will be ready for action."

What does Frank Sinatra sing that is sexy? The romantic mood he was trying to convey was not working. Martha and I laughed at him.

"Is it possible there was a mistake in the results?" I asked.

Dr. Uro looked at the chart and asked, "You are Michael Honeycutt, aren't you? Is your birth date August 17, 1947?

"Yes, to all," I said.

"Then these results are yours."

"When you did the biopsy, three of the slices were cancerous. These have been cut open. Will the cancer cells spread to other parts of the body by the opening in the prostate from the biopsy? I think of it as having a cut. The opening releases blood. Does opening a cancerous place allow it to get out of some enclosed and confined area?" I asked.

"That is a good question; the answer is no. The opened areas would not spread cancer through the body or into the bloodstream," he said.

"How many radical prostatectomies have you done?" I asked.

"Somewhere between two hundred and three hundred."

"I read most of Dr. Walsh's book. I learned a lot from this book. There seems to be a feeling that going to Johns Hopkins for this operation is safest. How much do I get from Johns Hopkins that is not available from the facilities here in Spartanburg?" I asked.

"We have as good a facility as any place in the world. If you would like to have another doctor review your case or do the operation, I am more than happy to help them in any way," he said.

"Last Sunday morning I thought about going to the Mayo Clinic. I went to their website and gave it some thought. Later in the day, I realized that this would not be a consideration. I know several people who had this surgery done by you. They are all pleased. You answered my question about your experience," I said. "How much better can a doctor get after doing over two hundred of these surgeries? How long do I have before I need the surgery?"

"Prostate cancer moves slow. You have time to make decisions and plans," he said.

"How long—a year?" I asked, smiling.

"Not that long." He smiled back. "You do need to wait six weeks for the biopsy to heal before surgery. I suggest some time shortly after the six-week period."

This did not make sense, but at least I had six weeks. We were going on vacation, so it would be after that time. I thought, *Now I must wait on my butthole to clear up before prostate surgery. A colonoscopy and biopsy were performed on me within four days of each other. I must wait on my rectum to rectify itself.*

"What happens during surgery?" I asked.

"First I suggest removing some lymph nodes and sending them to pathology. We can get a good determination from this if the cancer has escaped the prostate," he said.

"What if the lymph nodes show it has escaped the prostate?" I asked.

"We do not remove the prostate. There is no need. We then proceed with treating the cancer within your body. But, looking at your report, this should not be a concern. I am very sure we have caught this in time, and it is confined to the prostate,"

"After surgery what happens as far as recovery?"

"In surgery you will have a catheter inserted," he said. "During the healing process, this tube will make sure the urethra track does not close up. After surgery, we want to get you up and walking as soon as possible. It is important to get you walking quickly. The exercise is needed to get the body to overcome incontinence. Walking will be key in recovery. It is very important to walk and do as much as you can each day."

"How many days in the hospital?"

"About three; maybe four," he said.

"What do we do next?"

"You need to schedule a time for the operation. We have a staff person who schedules these for us. I will introduce you to her, and you can call back later when you decide," he said.

"I guess that's about all we have to ask presently," I said.

"Please call me anytime. I know his is very difficult for you. Remember, if we get the prostate out with a hundred percent of the cancer confined, you are cancer-free. Many people with other types of cancer do not have that possibility. If you were diagnosed with lung cancer, you would be in surgery immediately to remove all or part of the lung. The chances of it not spreading are very slim," he said. "We do not need to be overly concerned with all the options and all that could possibly happen. You will do fine. Do not get involved with every possibility. We need to take this one step at a time. Once we complete one process, we will then know what our options are for the next step. You will be back to your current physical condition in four or five weeks. You may even show an improvement in your physical condition. With this type of surgery, you will not lose your appetite," he said.

One of the nurses who had wished me well came over to me and said, "A gentleman is here who was recovering from the surgery and wanted to tell you something. He said the hardest part was the removal of the catheter after two weeks, which turned out to be a piece of cake."

I thanked her. Dr. Uro agreed and said this person was quickly recovering.

We left and had some simple conversation in the car on the way home. At home Martha did exactly what I wanted her to do—she was positive and got started on what we should do. We thanked God it was detected early and did as much as we could to prepare for surgery and recuperation. Martha said she was not leaving the hospital until I checked out.

CHAPTER 17

PLANNING WHAT TO DO

Martha and I left for vacation. We had made those reservations months in advance and were looking forward to getting away. We did have some decisions to make. We were to contact Dr. Uro's office and discuss the dates for the operation.

Our vacation was at a resort in the mountains in Massanutten, Virginia. The weather was great. This place had all types of activities.

We went scuba diving and canoeing and took water aerobics and exercise classes. One day we visited some wineries in the area. The wine tasting was fun and educational. All the wineries gave us tasting glasses. One had the following imprint:

US Army, be all you can be…
Bill Clinton, get all you can get…

One evening we had a wine tasting dinner. Wine was served with each course. A representative from the winery explained each type of wine and why it was provided with each course. This was nice.

There were four couples at our table. One couple was of Asian descent. I enjoyed talking to them. It was fun listening to their accents and discussing their vacation. I had met them earlier in the week. Another couple was from Harrisburg, Pennsylvania. I talked to them about the annual Little League Baseball World Series held in Harrisburg. Hearing about how the city prepared and all the volunteer work involved was interesting. The last couple was from New Jersey. They were very entertaining. The wife was what I call typical New Jersey. They had their four-month-old baby with them. The wife was a lawyer and worked in the twin towers in New York. I often think about the possibility of her having been there during 9/11. I think about the young child and pray she was not there on that day.

Scuba diving was fun. We were in one of the indoor pools, and space was a problem. After the training, we were to go underwater and practice. Martha could not do it and got out of the pool. She was afraid of the equipment and trying to breathe through the air tank line. A young boy, a young man, and I threw things to each other underwater. It was like Frisbee. The young boy really enjoyed that we let him participate. If Lloyd Bridges saw me, he would have been proud. All I knew about scuba diving came from watching the television series *Sea Hunt* staring Lloyd Bridges.

One afternoon Martha had a body massage. She loved it and wanted me to have one. I was waiting for her in the lobby when she finished. She came out and started telling me all about it. I was impressed and desired to have a massage.

"Did you have a man?" I asked.

"No, I would not feel comfortable with a man giving me a massage unless it was you," she said.

"I would not feel comfortable with a man giving me a massage," I said. "In fact, I will not do it."

"Then get a woman. You should have one; it's great," she said.

I was surprised she suggested I get one with a woman. I think she felt so good from the massage, and she just wanted to share that feeling with me. I talked with the girl who gave Martha her massage. She was a slim young girl with a Southern accent. After the discussion about a massage, she started talking about having a problem with one of her teeth. She told me her symptoms. I told her she probably needed a root canal. She expressed her fear of dentists. I tried to explain that a root canal is not painful. I told her that I had had two of them, but I do not think I convinced her. She said she was not going unless she absolutely had to.

I walked over to the receptionist's desk to make an appointment. The young girl making the reservations and answering the telephone had a pierced tongue. She had this silver ball in the middle of her tongue. I was surprised at the size of the hole through her tongue. I began to question her about it as though I liked it. I also boosted her confidence by bragging about how brave she was by doing it. She told me it did not hurt. She was a friendly person with a bubbly personality who could carry on a decent conversation. Surely, she will grow out of this and remove the silver ball from her tongue.

The next day I arrived for my massage. I spoke with the receptionist, and she asked me to have a seat. Someone would be with me shortly. A woman came out in a uniform like that of the slim young girl's outfit. This was not the slim woman with the southern accent, though. She was a strongly built woman from Russia. She introduced herself, and we shook hands. Those are firm hands, I thought. I was taken into a small, dimly lit room with a small-looking bed and pillow. Relaxing music played, and a lamp in the corner was the only light. She asked me to lie face down. Her accent was interesting, but because of it, she did not seem friendly. I quickly realized I was wrong. She was nice and asked me questions that relaxed me. She was very good. She'd completed her training in Los Angeles, not Russia. She stated that the best professional schools for massage are in Russia and that she wished she'd attended one of them. Her husband was trained in Russia. They met in Los Angeles. He was in the next room, massaging a man.

I admit it did feel a little strange when she announced her husband was in the next station, and I could hear his voice. I have absolutely no idea why I felt that way, but it probably had something to do with me lying on a bed in a closed, dimly lit area with a strange woman's hands on me.

We were to call Dr. Uro's office in the middle of the week to get some possible dates for my surgery. It was midmorning when we called his office. We were coming from the swimming pool. We sat down on a picnic table in the shade, and I called Dr. Uro's office on my cell phone. I asked to speak with the woman Dr. Uro introduced me to about scheduling the surgery. She gave me three dates. I said I wanted to discuss it with Martha and would call her back. She asked that I not wait too long because the dates would fill up quickly.

I was so thankful Martha recommended we do it as soon as possible. We had to wait six weeks after the biopsy. This date was right at six weeks. We all agreed on the last week in July for the operation. This was the earliest time available. By the time the day came for surgery, I was tired of waiting.

I brought two books with me on our vacation: *The Prostate*, by Dr. Patrick Walsh, MD, and Janet Farrar Worthington, and *No Such Thing as a Bad Day: A Memoir*, by Hamilton Jordan. I started reading them before we went on vacation. I wanted to study them and let Martha read them. She said she could not read them.

When we returned from vacation, I decided that I would take Hamilton Jordan's advice and get in the best shape possible. I started jogging and walking. I started working out at Gold's Gym. I was doing body pump and spin classes.

Before my surgery, I had to give two pints of blood. This blood was to be available during the surgery in case I needed it. I went to the blood bank downtown to give my first pint. I had a sheet of paper stating that I was to give blood for myself. The receptionist did not understand at first. After we figured it out, she led me to a small office.

Another woman came in and introduced herself. "I need to get a sample of blood," she said. "If the count is low, we will have to wait another day to take a pint."

She pricked my finger. The blood went up into a very small vial.

She came back a few minutes later and said it was fine for me to donate a pint of blood and to follow her. She led me to a large room with several couches and asked me to sit down.

Another woman came up, introduced herself, and applied a tourniquet. She inserted the needle. It was very smooth. She and I talked briefly. I was impressed with her; we got along well. She told me they could save blood for up to twenty-eight days. After a brief time, she came over and measured the amount of blood in the pouch and removed the needle. She offered me a drink of juice or cola and asked me to sit for a few minutes in case I felt dizzy.

I politely declined a drink and sat there for a few minutes even though I was feeling fine. I got up and did feel a little faint, but not enough to sit back down.

I returned to work and took it easy for the rest of the day. I did not exercise that day.

The next day I started exercising again. I tired easily. Assuming it was from the blood donation, I was not concerned. Each day I was less tired and felt better.

I went back to the blood bank again the next week. I did not get the woman I had last time and was disappointed. I saw her, and she nodded at me as if she recognized me.

This woman was nice, but the insertion of the needle was not as smooth. We did not have the conversation like I had had with the other woman.

When it was over, she offered me a drink. I felt a little woozy and took a coke. I relaxed and drank the coke. When I got up, I felt a little dizzy but was fine to drive.

The next day I started to exercise, but I decided not to go to Gold's Gym. I would walk and jog around the block. I did not get very far and returned home. The same thing happened the next day—I was totally weak and tired. I had to give up on exercising. The loss of two pints of blood in two weeks was making me very weak. No wonder they make you wait approximately a month between donations of blood.

I was also given a prescription for antibiotics. These were to be taken a week before surgery. The antibiotics also made me feel weak.

CHAPTER 18
SURGERY

After the surgery I will not need a digital rectal exam ever again, I thought. Anyone living in America has heard stories about this procedure. Most are hilarious. Some of the ones I've heard still make me laugh.

Martha and I were scheduled for a pre-op meeting at the hospital a day or so before the surgery. During the meeting we were told when to arrive, what to expect, what to wear, and all sorts of things patients and relatives need to know.

The night before surgery was lonely. I wanted tomorrow to be over. We had to get up at 5:00 a.m. and be at the hospital at 6:00 a.m. I was weak from the blood loss and antibiotics I was on. Martha was very careful with her words. She kept assuring me everything would be all right. After tomorrow it would be over, and she and I would start the recovery. I did sleep well. I was mentally and physically exhausted.

The next morning, we arrived at the hospital. I went into the receptionist's office with Martha. The woman told me I had to be shaved. I would then return to a waiting room.

I went into a room where another woman shaved me with an electric razor all over the penile area. She and I talked as though we were acquaintances. She was from Gaffney, and I knew her husband. It was sort of embarrassing, but at that point, I didn't have much concern about what was going to be done to me. After the loss of blood, the antibiotics, the early-morning awakenings, and having major surgery, what did I care if some strange female shaved my balls? She was just doing her job. An erection never occurred to me. Just another day at the barbershop.

When I left the room, I opened the wrong door. I saw a guy I knew from riding motorcycles. We knew each other by face, but not by name. We spoke for a minute. He was looking for his daughter who had wandered away. He was there for back surgery.

I found my way back to the waiting area where Martha and my son Michael were. We waited with the other people who were having surgery and their family and friends. All of us had the same feelings about not knowing what was next or when we would be called. I wasn't quite sure what to say.

They called my name, and we got up and walked down a hall. I went into a room and was told to put on my gown. *I might as well buy one of these things,* I thought. The woman said this would be the last time I saw Martha and Michael until I woke from the surgery. It was a short wait before they came and got me. We kissed and said goodbye.

"Don't let them castrate you," Michael said.

I climbed onto a gurney and was rolled into a large room with lots of lights. It was cold in the room. There were several people moving around and talking, all of them wearing green scrubs. Most of them wore sweatshirts of diverse types underneath the green smocks.

Dr. Uro told me later that we talked, and the last thing I wanted was for him to remove some lymph nodes for evaluation. I did not remember this. He told me later, after the surgery, that when they got to the point of removing the lymph nodes, he had an unobstructed view of the prostate and was sure we had caught it early enough. He started not to remove the lymph nodes but did so because that was the last thing I told him. He said he would wait on the results but felt there was no need to.

While I was in surgery, Martha and Michael had some people in the waiting room with them. Debbie Lyles, my brother Brian, my dad, and Martha's brother J. V. were there. Interestingly my dad's former neighbor, who was my high school football coach, was also there. His wife was having surgery. J. V. told me later that Martha was a strong woman.

Every so often they would call to the waiting room and give Martha an update on the surgery. The second time they called Martha, she went into a small glass-covered room and took the telephone call. Michael was there with her, and Brian was standing in the doorway. While she was talking, everyone in the waiting room could see her on the telephone. The nurse was telling her that everything was fine, but for some reason, she broke down and started crying. Everyone looking became nervous, thinking she had received terrible news. She came out and said, "Everything is going great. I don't know why I just broke down and started crying."

She sat down, everyone consoled her, and she felt better. Brian leaned over and told her, "You scared the crap out of me."

CHAPTER 19

AFTER SURGERY

In my mind I was going to cooperate with the nurses and doctors during my stay in the hospital. I wanted to be the perfect patient.

My first encounter with a nurse was a problem. She kept getting things confused. She did not bring me anything I asked for. She seemed unable to find anything. I noticed she had something written on her badge referring to being a temporary employee, and I thought all those bad things I heard about hospitals were true.

I never saw her again. All the other nurses I had were great. They knew what they were doing and were helpful and friendly. I knew the stepfather of one of them. Martha was always politely asking them for something and they would get it.

Everyone encouraged me to get up and walk. This was always part of any conversation with a nurse, a doctor, or Martha. I did get up to walk the first time I was supposed to, and it was not too bad. It wasn't so much tiring as it was an effort to be coordinated. Every time I was supposed to get up and walk, I did. It was good for me, and I really put forth an effort. Martha was always encouraging me and helping me get up out of the bed. I had her bring my darkest sunglasses so I could wear them when I made my rounds and while in bed. The nurses smiled.

I had some occurrences of bad headaches. I had a couple of these headaches in the hospital, and light made it worse. Neither aspirin nor Advil helped. My internist later diagnosed them as migraine headaches. This was the reason for my wanting those dark sunglasses. When I had those severe headaches, I wore the sunglasses, turned out lights, and closed all the blinds, but nothing really helped.

It was great to get visitors. They made me feel better, and I was happy for Martha when they came. It helped with the long hours. The only problem with visitors was they made me very tired. One day I had four different sets of visitors. The last were my friends, Big O and Amis. They are always great to listen to and would tell me something funny all the time. I was so tired that night. I made a comment that I was tired, and they got the message and left. They are good people to be around.

I woke up one afternoon, and a man who was mostly bald and wearing an Episcopal priest collar was looking at me. Briefly, in my drowsiness, I thought God had sent him to get me. Then he told me who he was, and I recognized him. He was the priest at the Church of the Incarnation, the episcopal church in Gaffney. We had a good chat; it was good to see him.

Another visitor was one of the priests, Father Brown, from the Episcopal Church of the Advent in Spartanburg. We talked, and then he asked, "Could we pray together?"

"Sure—you could pray with me, you can pray for me, but I'm not ready for you to pray over me," I said.

He laughed, and the three of us prayed together.

Dr. Uro came by and announced, "Your pathology results from the removed prostate were excellent. All indications show that the cancer was caught early enough. It should be confined in the prostate. No need to think about radiation around the area where the prostate was located."

This was the first time I'd heard about the possibility of radiation treatment around the area where the prostate was located. I did remember this being done to my dad after surgery as an outpatient, but I did not ask why they did it to him. But the doctor explained that if any of the cancer is near the outer edge of the prostate, they do radiation on the area around where the prostate was. *Another bullet dodged,* I thought. I did not like the idea of not being told this was a possibility. Later, I remembered Dr. Uro telling me we needed to take this one step at a time and not be concerned about all the possibilities. He always stated that we needed to work on each stage as it came.

People sent me cards, flowers, and plants. On checkout day, Brian came by at lunch. He and Martha carried two plants to her car. He complained, "They ought not to allow people to send plants to patients in the hospital. If they do send them, they should be the ones to come and take them out to the car." These were heavy plants.

After I checked out, they rolled me out in a wheelchair, and Martha brought the car up to the exit. A young girl rolled me around to the side of the car. The wheelchair began to lean toward the car because of the downward slope of the ramp. She could not stop it from swinging around and bumping into the side of our car. It left a vertical dent about six inches long. I realized it could not have been avoided. Besides, who cares; I was going home. She and Martha got me in the car, and off we went.

Our friend Pam said her father had the same operation and recommended I get a bucket to hold my urine pouch. This was a great idea. Martha got me a blue bucket that I carried with me everywhere. Martha named it Ole Blue. It really was helpful because the pouch broke at the seam and began to leak. Thanks to Pam and Ole Blue, we did not have a big yellow stain on our bedroom carpet.

Martha went to find another urine pouch, but had trouble locating one. When she did find one, it was expensive and took her several hours. She was not happy about this search.

Walking around the neighborhood, I always had Ole Blue in my hand. People passing by in a car saw me standing or walking with a blue bucket in my hand. If they looked closely enough, they would see the tube coming out from my shorts into the bucket. I always felt funny when a car would pass me. I doubt if anyone could see the tube, but I just had this feeling that perhaps they knew my condition.

After waking from the surgery, I realized that there was a tube coming from inside my body out through my penis. Some questions began to surface. How did they get that big tube up inside this little hole? How far up inside me is this tube? How does it stay in there and not come out? Why is it done? How come it doesn't hurt as much as I thought it would? Has anyone ever had this tube inserted while awake? If they tried that on me, I would pass out. How much will it hurt when they take it out? Can I be put to sleep to have it removed? I might want to put a bullet between my teeth and bite down when they remove it. Is it one big yank, or do they do it slowly? Can I make that decision? Do I have to grunt and squeeze my buttocks to help in the removal? Do they dispose of them after removing, or, do they wash them and use them again on someone else?

The tube's purpose was to prevent the urethra tract from closing. Without the tube, the area where the surgery was performed could close. If that tract closed, I guess one would pee out of his mouth, nose, or ear. It would be hard to urinate out of the ear and hit the toilet. The tube is supposed to stay in for ten to twelve days. One of my friends had a reaction to the tube once and it was removed after eight days.

There was no pain with the tube and pouch; it was just a pain to move it around whenever I moved in the bed. Finally, I implemented a procedure: during the day, the tube lay over the top of my right leg. At night, I moved it under my leg. Putting it under my leg gave more length to the pouch, which was residing within the confines of Ole Blue. This allowed me to roll over with less movement from the pouch and tube.

An added accessory was a much smaller tube connected to a small pouch that had a Velcro strap around it. By removing the standard system and installing the smaller system, I could strap the pouch to my leg and walk around without Ole Blue. I used this several times when we went out in public. It was convenient.

My walking was good. The big problem was the heat. It was August and very hot, and I could not stay in the heat too long.

The day came to have the tube removed. I was very nervous. During our meeting with Dr. Uro, he told Martha, "Look at him; he is nervous about having this removed. We need to put him in a soundproof rubber room when the nurse takes it out."

They laughed, and I giggled. It was a funny comment except for the last part. The nurse is going to take this out? Wait a minute. This thing has shrunk so much; I don't want anyone to see it. It might be OK for the doctor to remove it, but a female nurse? I'd rather take some scissors, cut the tube off at the end of my penis, and leave it in me for the rest of my life. I felt like George Costanza on *Seinfeld*: "Do women know about shrinkage?"

Dr. Uro escorted me to the room. I thought he was kidding me when he said a nurse and he would do it. He smiled and said the nurse would be in shortly, and I could relax. I assumed he was going to get some tools and maybe a nurse to help him. Sure enough, in came a female nurse who said she would remove the tube. After wiping the perspiration from my forehead, I thought, *What the heck. I bet it'll give her something to talk about over dinner tonight with her husband.* "This guy is as close to having an inverted penis as humanly possible."

I stood up at her suggestion. I had not noticed before, but there was a small exit from the tube near my penis. She inserted a needle into this exit. Some liquid came out into the syringe and into a small pan she was holding. When all this liquid came out, I felt some pressure release from inside me. She told me this inflated the inside end of the tube to keep it in my bladder. This is what kept the tube inside me. Now that it was deflated, she could remove the tube.

Here it comes! My knees went weak; my heartbeat doubled. My forehead began to sweat again. *Brace yourself, Mike. Where is that silver bullet you were going to bring?*

"Are you OK?" she asked.

"Uh huh," I muttered.

She began to pull the tube out. It slid out as if it had Vaseline on it. No problem. No pain. It was not that long and did not hurt at all.

What a relief. This was the easiest part.

She asked me to go to the restroom and void my bladder. They wanted to make sure I could urinate without the tube and that there was no blockage.

"What if I can't?"

"Then we must reinsert the tube," she said.

My knees went weak, and my heartbeat doubled again. I slowly walked to the restroom. I closed the door and thought, "This better work."

Hallelujah! I can pee! Let the yellow stream flow!

Dr. Uro came around the corner as I was going back to the patient's room. He laughed and asked if it was as bad as I'd expected. I said no and told him about being able to void. We went into the room.

He gave me some instructions about trying to walk as much as possible. This would stop leakages. Then he told me about Depends. This had been mentioned before. Now he was suggesting

I get some and try them. Soon I could move on to a minipad. It would all depend on my progress.

We scheduled another visit, and I was off to the drugstore. We looked at the several types of men's diapers. I was in a hurry; I did not want to wet my pants while shopping. Martha bought the type she felt would be best for me.

The Depends felt awkward but not too bad. I felt secure wearing them. At least I felt no one would know when I had an accident. The Depends would absorb it and not show on my pants.

The first weekend after my operation, we went out to dinner with Brian and Maurine. We all sat around and told funny stories. At this stage in the recovery, I couldn't control my bladder when laughing. I felt secure wearing my Depends. Brian got up a couple of times to go to the bathroom during our dinner and conversation. The second time he got up, I asked, "Where are you going?"

"To the men's room."

"I've gone three times and don't have to get up from the table."

CHAPTER 20

REST AND RECOVERY

Martha and I were going to leave for the mountains as soon as the catheter was removed. This was for my recovery to relax and walk. It was much cooler in the mountains.

She packed up the car with little help from me. The house was all closed up. We got in the car, and off we went. I was excited about getting to our mountain home. Cooler weather and a laid-back atmosphere. Sitting on our deck looking at the mountain range is so relaxing.

We arrived in the mountains, and the weather was perfect. We relaxed. The temperature is approximately ten to fifteen degrees cooler than at home. I did my walking and really started to get my strength back.

One Sunday evening I was watching television, and Martha was on the telephone with our future daughter-in-law, Molly Beckenhauer. I heard this noise on our back deck. It sounded as if something was moving around back there—perhaps one of the lightweight deck chairs. This reminded me of an opossum who used to come into our garage and eat our cat's food. It would roll around the metal plate and make a loud noise.

I got up to go to the kitchen door with the intention of scaring away a raccoon or an opossum. The door was open. The screen door was closed. I looked out the screen door and directly into the face of a black bear. He stared at me just as I did him. He stood no more than four feet away from me, and the only thing separating us was a screen door. Though it was dark outside, his face was brightened by the kitchen light shining out through a window. His dark eyes focused on me. The shaft of his nose was brown, and his nostrils were black and opened wide. His mouth was closed. I will never forget the smell of this bear.

When I realized what I was looking at, I thought, *Oh hell.* My prayer was, "Please do not let me do anything to excite him. Mike, do not move quickly, no matter what he does."

We both stared at each other, waiting to see what the other was going to do. I knew if he decided to come at me, he would have had no problem. I realized my only chance was to grab the kitchen door and slam it on him if he charged me. I thought I better not slam the door unless he came at me. I would hope to get his foot or some body part caught between the door and the wall. Maybe that would hurt him enough to scare him off.

I do not know how long the stare down lasted. It felt like several minutes, but I'm sure it was less.

Looking at a bear's face this closely, without a cage separating us, gave me a cold feeling. The darkness of its face with the brown hair on its nose gave me the shakes.

Slowly, very slowly, I backed away from the door. Later, I felt as though that could have been a mistake. I was away from the door, prepared to slam it on him. If he had decided to come in, I could not have gotten away. I should have shut the door gradually.

I went into the room where Martha was and told her there was a bear on the deck. She told Molly about the bear and said she would call back later. We went back to the kitchen. Martha was moving fast to try to see the bear. She had no fear. When we looked out the door, the bear was gone.

We turned on the deck light, opened the door, and walked out. I saw why the bear was this close to the kitchen: it had been trying to get into a trash bag Martha had put out on the deck.

Martha went over to the steps that go up to the deck. We had a small gate to block the stairs and keep our dog from getting out.

"There has not been a bear here," she said.

"Why do you say that?"

"Because the gate is still blocking the steps up to the porch."

"He didn't use the steps. Come over here," I said.

The two-by-four banister was separated from the house and the post where it was mounted. He had climbed up to the highest part of the deck, about seven feet off the ground. We had a bird feeder hanging over the deck. The bear had climbed up the lattice sides and grabbed the bird feeder. When he got to the deck, he smelled the trash bag. This must have been a dessert tray compared to the birdseed. He must have carried the bird feeder with him. To this day, the bird feeder has never been found.

Martha believed me then. We both knew something strong or heavy had to separate that two-by-four from the house and post.

Martha called everyone we knew. There were others in our area who had seen the bear in the past; he had destroyed several bird feeders along our road.

The following is a letter I sent to my Sunday school class about this incident:

Dear Class,

Thank you for the card. It was really a pleasure to receive it and to hear from many of you.

My recovery improves daily. It seems to come in plateaus. My first plateau was going to the mountains where the temperature is about fifteen degrees cooler than home. I could do my walking.

My second plateau came one night when I heard noise on our deck, which is about seven feet above the ground. I walked into the kitchen and looked out the open door. I was looking directly at a black bear that also was staring at me. As the stare down continued, I remember my doctor gave me *strict orders* not to lift anything over ten pounds and not to move quickly. He did not mention it, but I am sure he did not want me wrestling with a black bear.

Realizing I must follow his *strict orders*, I decided Martha should protect us from this intruder. When I returned with her, the bear was gone.

Later that night we had to let our dog out. My first thought was to pitch the dog outside and slam the door, but I realized that he was a good friend, and because I was under *strict orders*, I decided Martha should walk him outside.

While watching Martha walk the dog, I decided I must protect my family. I found a poker iron for the fireplace and marched out the front door to guard my loved ones. I made loud noises by hitting the concrete porch floor with the poker iron. Remembering I was under *strict orders*, I stood one step away from the entrance, holding the door open in case I needed to get inside.

Thanks again for the cards and telephone calls. We miss all of you.

Sincerely,

Michael Honeycutt Sr.

The recovery in the mountains was wonderful. We had beautiful weather. Each day I increased my walking distance. I had switched to minipads. The Depends were no longer needed. I had started with the extra thick. This was a problem. I felt as though one could see a bulge in my pants, and the bulge did not look super manly in size. It looked like I had a small pillow in my underwear. It felt like I had a small pillow to lay my penis against. Anyway, I decided to switch to the thin ones.

Three people were really encouraging and helpful before and after my surgery. They told me about their experiences and what I could expect and helped to answer any questions I had. Each experience was different. For each one, a different doctor performed the procedure. They are all now patients of Dr. Uro. All of them were very positive about his abilities and the care he would provide. I am so thankful to them for offering their assistance.

After four weeks, I returned to work for half days. Martha made sure I left after a half a day. After a week I was back full-time.

As I began to get my strength back, a couple of things bothered me. Although my leakages were much better, it was not 100 percent. A quick movement would cause a dribble. When I went to work or out in public, the mini pads were on. A laugh would cause leakage. Sometimes if I moved my legs quickly some would leak out.

This got better with time, as predicted by Dr. Uro. I went cold turkey on the minipad one evening when we went to the movies. It was strange at first. I was proud of myself that evening and decided to forget those items.

Another problem was something I would describe as a spasm. This pain occurred in my crotch area. It really hurt, and I would have to lie down. We were scheduled to go out late one afternoon when I had one of these spasms. I told Martha about it and lay down. It eventually went away. The times I had these pains were when I had exceeded my normal amount of exercise or stood up for too long. They gradually came further and further apart, and eventually they went away.

If I had to compare this type of pain with something else, I would guess hemorrhoids. I'd never really experienced this type of pain before. I'd never had hemorrhoids, but the pain is close to that area of the body. Perhaps that's why I relate the two.

The big day came when I was scheduled to see Dr. Uro about a few things, one of which was having an erection. This subject is of utmost importance to men. Most men who have not had an elevated PSA—myself included—think of prostate removal as the end of the line for sex.

At approximately the fifth week after my surgery, I was working on my putting on the practice green. An old friend approached me, and the conversation went something like this:

"Hey, Mike. How are you doing?"

"I am doing well," I said.

"You look good. Have you started back playing golf?"

"No, just putting. If I swing a club, something might come undone," I joked.

"So how are you doing?" he asked, again.

"I am doing well. I started back to work last week."

"Well, can you get a hard-on?" he finally asked.

The last question was the first question he wanted to ask me. I knew it was coming from this guy. He has never been shy about asking anyone anything.

CHAPTER 21

MOVING FORWARD

I arrived and stepped into a private room at Dr. Uro's office and took note of what I was going to ask him. Most of my questions dealt with simple things that had occurred. Then I decided how to approach the question of an erection. *Do I bring the subject up as a question about having sex? Do I get directly to the subject and say I have not had sex? Do I just say I have not had an erection? I feel nervous talking to him about the subject. But other than Martha, he is the one person I feel most comfortable discussing these matters with. He knows all I have been through and what will be happening during my recovery. He probably has had this conversation thousands of times.*

Dr. Uro entered the room. We shook hands and exchanged some pleasantries. I mentioned golf, and he said he plays.

"Have you had an erection?" he asked.

"I woke up one night with a type of erection," I said.

"That's a good sign. Have you had any more?"

"No, I wanted to talk with you about that," I said.

"Your body has endured an enormous shock to its system. It will take time to overcome this. It may take up to one year. Just the trauma from the surgery takes a long time for your body to overcome. Therefore, we like to take things slowly and one step at a time. We have some methods to help you with an erection, if you're interested."

"Sure," I said.

"We can try Viagra," He said. "There is also the option of inserting a small tablet into the urethra tract, but I think the one we should try now is an injection. It's not as painful as you would initially think. One of my patients told me he wished he had known about this method many years ago. It is not painful, and you'll stay erect for a long time. You want to try this?" he asked.

"Where is this injection going to be?"

"In the penile area, but it will not hurt,"

"Yes, if you think this is the way to go," I said.

"Make an appointment to come back next week, and I will go through how this works. It won't take long to show you, and I promise it is not painful. You do the injection, put on some Frank Sinatra music, and in about ten minutes with some foreplay, it will "rise for the occasion."

There he goes with Frank Sinatra again.

I made an appointment on my way out for the following week. I wanted to do it that day, but he wanted to wait a week. Now I must think about this all week. I have already thought about this needle insertion many times. I hoped we would not go there.

Am I going to be able to do this to myself? Lots of people give themselves injections for diabetes. Yeah, but not where I get to shoot myself. I had a biopsy in the penile area once. They gave me a shot in the penis to numb the area, and it hurt.

I arrived at Dr. Uro's office for the training. I was sitting in the exact same patient's room where he told me I had prostate cancer. He came into the room with a pamphlet that explained the entire procedure. It had diagrams and all sorts of graphic designs. After the explanation, he reached into his lab coat and pulled out this blue plastic box. In it was a syringe and a small bottle. The syringe had some fluid inside; the bottle had powder.

He showed me how to insert the fluid from the syringe into the bottle. Shake it up. He informed me to always make sure it was a clear fluid.

"I recommend you get smaller syringes so you can get the correct amount needed. It will take a couple of times to get the correct dosage. Once you do, there may be enough left to use a second time. These kits are expensive. I doubt you will need the whole bottle.

"I will do the injection. There are two areas on top of the penis where there are very few nerves: they are on each side of the penis at the top. I suggest you rotate sides. Do it close to the body. Look at the skin, and avoid any blood vessels."

He inserted the needle. Strangely enough, there was no pain. In fact, I was concerned because there was no pain. He quickly pushed on the stem, and the fluid escaped the syringe. He removed the needle. I felt absolutely no pain at all.

"I am going to leave you here for about ten minutes. You should have an erection when I return. You can put your pants on. Just let me know if it works."

As I flipped through some magazines, sure enough, I started getting an erection. As it got bigger. I felt a small throbbing feeling, just enough to be noticeable.

When he came back into the room, he asked how I was doing.

"Fine," I said, "it works."

"Good. It will take about an hour for it to go away. You can go home or back to work—anything you feel like doing."

"I do have a small throbbing feeling," I said.

"It has been over two months since you've had an erection. That is to be expected. It is not a problem."

I drove back to work. In the office, I sat at my desk and did not get up. I was concerned someone would see me. It did feel funny. This erection lasted about an hour.

That evening Martha and I went to get the prescription for the injection filled. The first pharmacy had not heard of this prescription. The young technician asked the pharmacist, and he said they did not have it in stock. The same thing happened at the next pharmacy.

We went to BI-LO for some groceries. I went to the pharmacy section. The pharmacist was about my age. He looked at the prescription. He did not have it in stock, but he searched his computer to see if they could get a delivery. He said it would be several days and apologized. As I walked away, he called me back. "You might try Smith Drugs downtown. They carry all types of prescriptions."

Sex in the Honeycutt passion pit would have to wait another day. Maybe weeks. I may have to go to Mexico and smuggle this stuff in.

I went to Smith Drugs. This was an old pharmacy like I was used to when I was growing up. I liked the place. I was reminiscing about my younger days. An older man looked at the prescription. He did not carry it, but he could get some here in three days.

As I left, I kept thinking, no sex tonight. Where did Dr. Uro's patients get this prescription filled?

The next day Martha found a pharmacy that said they could have it here tomorrow. She told them to get some and that she would pick it up the next day.

The next day she picked up the prescription. The woman informed her they would stock it if we were going to have it refilled every so often. Martha gave her our prescription insurance card. She said our insurance did not cover this prescription. Five of these blue boxes were over one hundred dollars.

Martha called me at work and told me the news about insurance not covering the costs and how much she had to pay. *The price of sex just went up twenty dollars. Ah! The passion pit will be hot tonight.* I didn't care if it cost one hundred dollars per blue box.

Work went by slowly. I arrived home, and we prepared dinner. We were talking jokingly, excited about what was to come. Finally, the evening arrived. I was excited about having sex with my wife. I was also very nervous about using the needle.

I opened the prescription's paper box labeled "Cavaject for injection 20 micrograms." Inside were five blue boxes. The instructions had warning signs all through them. There was a red stub to insert in the box when finished so it could not be opened again. I assumed this was for safety reasons to keep someone from reusing the syringe. There was a small bottle with powder in it. The syringe contained a fluid, and the plunger was not inside the syringe.

I read the instructions. They were simple to read and very easy to follow. I remember Dr. Uro suggesting I find the correct amount to use and to buy some insulin syringes as small as you can get. Martha had bought a box of BD Ultra-Fine Needle Insulin Syringes. These are used by diabetics. There were one hundred in the box. How long would it take to use one hundred of these? I hope she looked for the expiration date.

First, I noted the instructions said to mix the fluid and powder and use only as much as needed. Do not save the remaining to use later. OK, I will throw away what I don't use until I talk with Dr. Uro again.

When Dr. Uro did the injection, he used 20 cc. That seemed to do the job. But I wanted to make sure. I loaded it up to 23 cc. I did not want the first time to be a "no-show." What can be the difference in 3 cc anyway?

I was in the bathroom behind closed doors doing all this. Martha was in the bedroom. She asked, "Is it working?"

"I just completed the instructions. I don't want to make a mistake. I must be careful and not overlook anything," I said.

The time had arrived. Instructions had been memorized. Martha was getting bored in the bedroom. Am I going to do this or not? No more stalling.

As I dropped my head to look down, I got dizzy. My hands started to shake. As I looked up into the mirror, I grinned at myself and thought, "another fine mess you're in." This calmed me down. Again, I looked down. I was not as dizzy.

Stretching out my penis with left hand, I looked for a place to insert the needle, which was in my right hand. The instructions said to look for a place where there were no blood vessels. I was to locate a place on the left or right side and not use the middle. This is hard to do at my age with my vision. I found a location that looked good. Putting the needle to my skin, I jumped nervously and let go with my left hand.

Damn! I had to start all over.

As I searched for the correct place to insert the needle and was just moving the needle in place, I heard "Is it working?" This scared me again.

"Not yet, but it will be soon," I said.

"Well, hurry up and get in here," she said. "Have you done it yet?"

"Not yet; I was ready when you interrupted me."

Third time's a charm, so they say. I stretched, inspected for blood vessels, put the needle to the skin, and pushed.

It's in there, and it doesn't hurt! Squirt the juice in and pull that thing out! No pain. Wow! This is not bad. I put my equipment on the vanity and danced into the bedroom.

"Stand back, baby, I don't know how big this thing is going to get! It may fill up one of your shoe boxes!" I was rocking and rolling. I dove onto the bed. We lay there, laughing, waiting for the erection. Martha made a comment about not having any Frank Sinatra music. Where did Dr. Uro come up with Frank Sinatra?

When our mission was complete, I assumed the erection would go away. It did with Viagra. Wrong—it stayed, pointing like a dog on the hunt. I finally got out of bed. As I walked, the weight of my erection pulled it down. It bounced up and down as I walked to the bathroom. *Now what?* I thought. *I guess I wait.*

I waited for about an hour. Finally, it began to recede. Man, what a difference 3 cc can make. It was so hard I don't think a cat could have scratched it. *Next time I will use less serum.*

Throughout the period of getting this process correct, I made some errors. It is best to get the correct amount of volume. Mine was about 21 cc. I do suggest the insulin needles. You can get a more accurate amount. The scale has larger print, and the diameter of the syringe is smaller. Both allowed for better accuracy.

Cavaject is also a viable alternative. It works well if you are careful and follow instructions.

CHAPTER 22
PSA < 0.1

Three months after my surgery was my first scheduled PSA. I stopped by Dr. Uro's office. I'd scheduled a visit to go over the results. I was sent to the bottom floor to a lab. They took my blood. The results would not be ready for about three days, which was my scheduled visit with the doctor.

On the day of my doctor's visit, I really expected the best. Why not? All the information given to me was excellent. The nurse sat me down and asked me a few questions about how I was doing. We talked for a few minutes, and then I asked, "Do you have the results of my PSA?"

She flipped through my file and said, "Yes. Your number is perfect."

She then led me down the hall to a private office. As I waited for the doctor, I looked around the room. Nothing seemed to have changed. There were several boxes containing tubes of K-Y Jelly. Hmm, he will not be using that on me ever again. The rubber gloves were in a box. *I am sure there will be a reduction in production of those things now that I have no prostate. I need to check the name of the company in case I own stock in it. If so, I better sell; their revenue will drop.*

Dr. Uro walked in with my file. He looked at the results and said, "The PSA was perfect. It was 0.01. This is as low as it can go."

"How does it feel knowing you had cancer and are now cancer-free?" he asked.

"Great!" I said.

This is what all cancer patients want to hear from their doctor. Early detection allows your doctor to say this to you. How many cancer patients would love to hear those words spoken to them? The risks associated with a radical prostatectomy are minimal compared with having prostate cancer spread.

I had not thought that much about it. I always felt that it was caught in time. If caught in time, none of the cancer escapes the prostate. The concern of all individuals diagnosed with prostate cancer is to stop the cancer cells from leaving the prostate. Prostate cancer is slow-moving. Once it escapes the prostate, it spreads to other parts of the body. The spreading is slow. The unfortunate thing is that, as the cancer spreads, the newly invaded parts of the body become very painful. It usually spreads to the bones. During the deterioration of the body from prostate cancer, the brain, lungs, and heart operate fine. You are alert and have feelings.

Dr. Uro talked a little about what I should be doing. He was happy to hear I was playing golf. He had returned my call a few weeks earlier. I was playing golf, and he spoke with Martha. He wanted me to continue to exercise and do whatever I wanted. I should be back to normal soon, if not already.

The next scheduled PSA was in three months. For the first year after surgery, a PSA checkup should be done every three months. After the first year, a PSA should be done every six months for the next five years. After that, who knows? I did not ask.

In October Martha and I attended TQCA's (Textile Quality Control Association) annual meeting in Myrtle Beach, South Carolina. This was an enjoyable time of year to visit Myrtle Beach. The weather was perfect.

It was good to see the members of this group. Several of them wanted to know how I was doing. Mrs. Kim, the executive secretary of the group, had kept in touch with me by telephone or e-mail. Kim was also employed by an organization that had scheduled me to present a paper. I chose to cancel and have the surgery. From my canceling the presentation, she knew what was going on. She was always helpful and very positive about my recovery. Her encouragement helped and will always be remembered.

We had a relaxing three days at Myrtle Beach. Martha and I enjoyed each other. We needed this getaway.

CHAPTER 23

BACK TO NORMAL

After full recovery, about forty-five days, it was highly recommended I have a PSA test every six months for the first two years; after that, once a year every year. If all the results were less than 0.02, the possibility of the cancer having been removed before escaping the prostate was great. I had cancer, and now I do not have cancer. Not remission—*gone*!

Should the PSA results show an increase over 0.1, there would be cause for concern. That is an episode I currently do not have to address.

I remember a comment by Richard Petty, the famous NASCAR driver. After getting PSA results with a low reading, he feels excited and wants to celebrate.

I totally agree.

CHAPTER 24

MICHAEL'S WEDDING

Our son Michael got engaged. This was great. He was dating Molly Beckenhauer. They met at Clemson University. Molly was from Martinez, Georgia.

On July 13, 2002, my son married Molly in Augusta, Georgia. The three days of this wedding were some of the greatest of our lives. My dad and I drove down to Augusta together. He was concerned about going; his health and being part of the wedding was a concern to him. Once he gets involved, though, he adapts very well.

The wedding was my first Catholic wedding. I was told it would be much longer than the typical weddings I had attended in the past. The church was magnificent. The service was great. I was so proud of Michael and all Molly and her family had done. Maurine sang a couple of solos. With the acoustics in the church, her voice was beautiful.

After the wedding, we were to drive to the reception. Molly got her wedding dress prepared for the reception, which meant removing part of it. There was no way she could get in a car wearing her entire wedding dress. Her sisters and mother worked on downsizing it.

Between the church and our wedding reception locations was another wedding reception. I think everyone attending our wedding on the groom's side went to this reception by mistake. Billy Osborne went in and had a drink in his hand before realizing he was at the wrong place. He figured it out when he realized the bridesmaids were wearing dresses that were different colors than the bridesmaids at our son's wedding. Mike Fleming stopped his car at the same place and let his wife, Julia, out. He drove around to the back to park the car, walked to the front, and went in to look for Julia. Julia noticed their mistake immediately and walked down the street to our reception without first locating Mike. He wasn't paying much attention to the people but eventually realized he was in the wrong place. After Mike decided Julia was not there, he got in his car and drove to our reception.

We had an exciting time at the reception. All the food was wonderful. The band was good. We danced and laughed. Martha and her group, the "inseparable six," started a dance to the song "Continental Walk." We lined up men on one side and women on the other, facing one another. The couple at the head of the group would dance down the line, strutting their stuff. All the dancers were lacking in all areas. Like the old saying goes, "Alcohol was invented so white people would get up and dance."

As the reception was about to close because we had to be off the premises at 1:00 a.m., I noticed the guys from Michael's rugby team headed out the door with a keg of beer. They were going to take it to their hotel and finish it. Dennis Beckenhauer, Molly's father, went over and stopped them. He spoke to them briefly. They all cheered and went off with the keg.

Back at our hotel again, we gathered at the bar. It was packed. A convention had just started that day—the National Wild Turkey Federation. Turkey calls were used to let the waitresses know it was time for another drink. I tried a turkey call and was booed.

CHAPTER 25

NINETY-DAY COMPETITION

I was looking forward to returning to Gold's Gym to start working out.

One evening as I was walking out, someone said, "Excuse me, sir. Did you have a good workout?"

"Yes, what is it you're promoting with your table display?" I asked.

"Why do you come here to work out? What are you trying to accomplish?" he asked.

"I want to lose this inner tube around my waist," I said.

"You need to burn more calories and eat fewer fat and carbohydrates," he said. "Most Americans eat over two hundred to three hundred grams of carbohydrates a day. If you reduce that to less than a hundred a day and continue to exercise, you will lose your stomach. One of our products is low in fat and carbohydrates and high in protein. Taking this with water or milk will fool your stomach. There will be food there, and you will not have an appetite. Your body will need to burn your body fat for energy because you have not eaten fat or carbohydrates. This will allow you to lose body fat faster."

"Let me have the literature. I have to evaluate what ingredients are in these vitamin supplements and protein drink," I said.

I went on the company's website and learned about their program. For two weeks I thought about trying it. Their exercise program and diet recommendation made sense. I was still concerned about taking supplements, especially high-protein supplements. Protein has been referred to as the culprit for my gout and kidney stones.

Before my biopsy, I began noticing it was taking me longer to get warmed up before exercising. I was having problems walking when I first got out of bed each morning or if I sat for very long. I became stiff. Just before surgery it had gotten bad.

I felt very stiff in my ankles and legs from sleeping or sitting for periods of time. Both of my shoulders in the deltoid area were always stiff. Sometimes at the gym, they never loosened up. I had to scale back on the amount of weight I was lifting. By the time surgery came, I was ready to quit.

I decided I would stop working out and start back after my recuperation. This would give my muscles time to get rid of this stiffness.

The second day in the hospital after surgery, I noticed the soreness was gone. This made me feel good. I had rested enough, and my muscles would allow me to start exercising again.

Two weeks after my surgery, this stiffness began to come back in my shoulders. It wasn't as bad, but it was back, and I was not exercising those muscles.

Six weeks after surgery, I visited Dr. Intern. I told him the story about my stiffness, how it went away after my surgery and came back a few weeks later.

He said, "Then you have arthritis. The body reacted to your surgery. It started developing steroids because of the trauma your body was going through. This was why your arthritis went away briefly.

"We can run all types of tests on you, but I do not think it's necessary. I can send you to specialists, and they could run all types of tests, but they will treat you the same as I will.

"This is a prescription for Vioxx," he said. "It will help you. Then we can go from there. Arthritis is very unpredictable. It could get better or worse. It could even go away. But if it doesn't get worse, this might be enough. If it gets worse, I'll send you to a specialist."

The Vioxx did help me. It reduced my stiffness. I was having problems moving my arms and legs without a concentrated effort. In a car, if I had to reach around my shoulder to get my seatbelt, it was a concentrated effort to reach around with my right hand to grab it. It felt like my arms weighed much more than normal.

Reading about Vioxx and NSAIDs was encouraging. These types of drugs are helpful for pain. They are long lasting and not as bad for your stomach as previous types of prescription drugs or aspirin. However, there is a warning that continued use might be harmful to the stomach.

I used Vioxx for an abbreviated period and began to feel better. The stiffness was going away. I began skipping days intentionally. Some days I could tell the difference, and some days I could not.

After a week of thinking about this young fellow promoting his products, exercising routinely, and dieting, I saw him at Gold's Gym again. We talked. I had considered the ingredients and was fine with what little I knew. He gave me the promotion speech again. We talked about a ninety-day competition program they were doing nationally as well as one specifically for the members of our gym.

This was a program designed to lower the percentage of body fat. The winner at our gym would have a choice of a Jet Ski or an ATV. All one had to do to enter the competition was buy more than one hundred dollars' worth of products and use them.

I decided to join the competition. Martha took pictures of me in my gym shorts. We were going to select one as my before photo. The date was on the photo. That evening when I went to Gold's Gym, I told Brad, the manager, that I wanted to enter the competition.

Brad sold me the products he thought I needed. We went into the locker room, and he took a Polaroid of me with the products. We went to his office, where I was measured and weighed. He measured my waist and arms. He took some measurements with calipers around my body. All these measurements were recorded. We talked for a few minutes. He recommended I take three lessons from one of the personal trainers. There would be no charge. He recommended another guy named Eisenhower.

The lessons were intended to get me familiar with the different machines. Once I was familiar, the personal trainer gave me some specific exercises I might want to use in my program. Some of them were machine exercises, while others required free weights.

I was ready to start. I had a diet, an exercise program, and supplements. At last I could lose weight. At home, I put a sticky note on my mirror and wrote the number ninety in the top-left corner. Each day I marked through the last number and wrote in the next number less one. This was my way of counting down the ninety days. It really helped me make it through.

I worked hard at the gym. I did as much aerobics as I could at each workout. Two days a week, I did a cycle class. This entailed riding a stationary bicycle for forty-five minutes with an instructor and music. This was a great workout that burned a lot of calories. It was the hardest of my aerobic workouts. In the later part of my training, after cycling, I would get on the elliptical machine and rode for over a mile.

After about thirty days or so, I decided to stop taking my allopurinol medicine. Allopurinol reduces uric acid in the blood. My uric acid started getting high about five years earlier. Previously, whenever I tried to stop taking allopurinol, I would have a gout attack or kidney stones. Each time I promised to never stop taking the medication. Both of those problems are very painful, to put it mildly. To this day, I have not a kidney stone. Twice I have had physicals, and my uric acid level has been below normal. I have had some minor gout attacks.

Sometime around the fifty-day point of my competition, I decided to stop taking Vioxx. After a couple of days, I was sure I needed to go back on the medication, but I didn't. I did not feel stiff or sore. As the days went by, I experienced no symptoms of arthritis. On occasion, I would take a Vioxx because of a headache or a muscle pain, but I have never gone back to Vioxx on a regular basis.

Everything I have read about arthritis suggests that exercising can be a major help. What one eats also has an effect. This has really been true for me. I can tell if I go for several days without exercising.

On days after consuming a few beers or a couple of glasses of wine, I can feel stiff and sluggish. Overeating is another way to get stiff and sluggish. After a workout or two, the symptoms go away.

Now I never get up in the mornings stiff. The stiffness doesn't bother me. Exercise is an effective way to overcome the type arthritis I have. However, I must refer to Dr. Intern's comments that it could go away for no specific reason.

Although I stayed on a diet, this was the hardest part. The protein drinks to help eliminate my hunger pains were a good idea in addition to eating good-quality foods and reducing my carbohydrate and fat intake. I did have some "cheat days," some of them concurrently. Each time I looked in the mirror and saw my sticky note, it helped me get back on the diet. It was a reminder that I was reducing the days and I needed to stick with it.

The time was getting close to the end of my ninety-day competition. What was I going to do about my after picture? I read something about how to pose for photographs that showed improvement for after pictures. We could submit our own photos along with the ones Brad had taken. I wanted to look good. Some of the suggestions were to have a light background. Wear dark clothing to contrast. Stand erect with shoulders back and abdomen squeezed in. Get a tan.

Get a tan? I have had two skin cancers removed from my face. My dermatologists said to be very careful in the sun. Always wear sunscreen and a hat, and no sunbathing. My skin is as white as the underside of a killer whale. I might not do the tanning part.

One Saturday I went to a pharmacy looking for lotions that promoted a tan without sun. I remember in high school there was something on the market called QT, which I believe stood for Quick Tan. All you did was rub it on, and the next day you had a tan. I was going to find QT and try that maybe. I did not find QT, but there were several other brands. Reading all the brands made me decide not to do this. There was too much time involved with waiting on the lotion to dry. I was also concerned about my hands turning orange, especially around the fingernails.

I changed my mind about a tan. Maybe just a little tanning bed time. Three weeks before my competition ended, I paid a monthly fee to use the tanning beds at the gym. I was not going to burn. I was going to go slow and gradually increase the amount of time in the tanning bed. I was going to keep my face covered. I used the tanning bed about eight times. It did feel good. I could tell a difference. While I was going to the tanning bed, I slipped around Martha. She would not be happy about me doing this.

I started making jokes to some of the people in the gym about using a tanning bed. One of the girls, Tanner, who'd also entered the ninety-day competition, always had a tan. One day before using the tanning bed, I told Tanner, "Look at my tan. I have been using those tanning beds for two months. Do you think it's working?"

"You need to get your money back," Tanner said, laughing.

"Well, to tell you the truth, I did not know you had to turn on the lights in the tanning bed. I was getting in there and lying down with no lights on. Then one day, I saw someone in there with the lights on and asked what the lights were for."

"Then you really need to get your money back," she said. I think she believed me.

There was one other recommendation to consider: shaving my body hair. How am I to do this? What parts am I going to shave?

Off again to a pharmacy. This time I was looking for something like Nair—just wipe on this cream, and wipe off the hair. I heard about waxing the hair off. I was amazed at all the different things available for hair removal. Not only was there Nair but several other brands to remove hair. Waxing must hurt. That was out.

I chose some brand that rolled on. The instructions said to leave it on for three to five minutes and wipe off the cream in a circular motion. The hair will come off with the cream. Yeah, right. I put some on a small area of my arm just above the wrist in the parking lot of this pharmacy. After five or so minutes, I pulled my truck over to side of the road. With my handkerchief, I removed the cream. I looked at my arm. It did not look as though any hair was gone. I looked at my handkerchief, and there was a lot of hair on it. Some did come off, but not enough to tell by looking at my arm.

I returned home, and Martha was gone. Now was my chance to shave. I had a small electric shaver I used to remove the hair on my neck. I started with it on my chest. This was easy to do. After I finished my chest, the view in the mirror showed hair around my stomach area. I shaved this and then went to the arms and then the fingers. The mirror showed me several other areas I needed to shave: the back of my arms, the tops of my shoulders, and around my navel. I shaved it all.

Baldness is loss of hair on the head. We refer to it as losing your hair. This isn't the case. The hair growth leaves the head and moves to other parts of the body. It comes up in the ears. It grows on the tops of shoulders. The arms get thicker.

Oh man! What have I done? This looks worse than I'd imagined. I'd had visions of looking like some of the bodybuilders who shave. The problem was my fifty-five-year-old skin. I'd hardly done anything for my skin. Rarely did I put on any lotion; why would I look like those bodybuilders? I was going to hide this from Martha.

That was it. I would not go for the legs. That's too much. And I sure am not going for the pubic area. No need to do the back either.

I was embarrassed. How long before this will grow back? People say it is very itchy to shave and let the hair grow back. Some say to keep powder on the area to help with the itching.

Finally, my ninety days were up. I wanted to put the measurements off a day because I thought I had retained too much water. But I had to do it on the last day. I decided I would never be ready and to go ahead and do it on the last day instead of waiting one more day.

Brad measured me. I had lost 8 percent of my body fat, ten pounds, and one and a half inches off my waist. My arms had increased almost a half an inch. He took my picture.

He complimented me and said I did well.

"Has anyone else finished the competition?" I asked.

"Yes, there were a couple of women. You are the first man," he said.

"I send the results off to D&A's corporate office. They do the judging," he said.

The competition I just completed answered any questions I had about being physically fit after a radical prostatectomy. I was in the best physical condition I had been in for over twenty years. This helped me overcome some episodes of depression I'd been having since the surgery. I felt good about myself. At times, I even thought I had a chance of winning the local competition.

One day after the competition, I walked in to Gold's Gym to work out. Brad asked to speak to me.

"We have been running ads in the newspaper showing before and after pictures of some of our members. Would you allow us to use your photos in our ad?" he asked.

"Sure. I would be glad to help."

"Have you seen the one ad we ran with Tanner?"

"Yes, I saw it. I was impressed with how much weight she lost," I said.

"Tomorrow we are running another with Tamera in it," he said. "I want to do one with a man's pictures. You did well, and your photos are great. I need you to write a small comment about why you did it or how you did it. I will help you."

"OK, go ahead; I know I will have fun with this," I said.

"Thanks; it will be in next Tuesday's paper. Watch for it."

Throughout that workout, I was on cloud nine. I repeated my conversation with Brad during dinner.

"I don't think so," Martha said. "I am proud of you, but I don't want other women seeing you posing."

I did not have the heart or nerve to tell her I had already given the go-ahead.

Next Tuesday morning, I went out to get the paper, and while thumbing through it, I found the ad. It was a two-column ad and not very noticeable. Maybe Martha wouldn't see it.

She did not see it, but one of her friends did and called her. They thought it was good, but Martha did not appreciate it. I showed it to her. She got a little mad but realized it was such a small ad that not many people would see it.

The next day at the office, our insurance agent Mike came by for a visit. He went on a diet several months earlier and had lost a lot of weight. After we talked insurance, he pulled out the picture in the paper. We laughed and talked about our accomplishments. After he left the office, I saw the ad on our bulletin board in our kitchen. I assumed he had put it there.

One our friends, Amy, cut it out and put it on her refrigerator. I got several compliments. Martha got some compliments, too, but she was not impressed.

On Wednesday, when I went into Gold's Gym, Brad and Darren were at the front counter.

"Fellas, I will be leaving Spartanburg soon," I said.

They looked at me for an explanation.

"I will be going to New York and Paris to pursue a modeling career. Telephone calls are already coming in from agents wanting to represent me."

"Yeah, sure," they said and laughed.

A couple of weeks later, Brad asked me if he could run the ad again.

I said, "Sure. I am enjoying the stardom."

"Thanks. It will be in Sunday's paper."

Sunday is the big day for reading the paper. Now this is going to be interesting.

I opened the Sunday paper, thumbed through it, and there it was. This was a bigger ad—a longer one that spanned three columns. It was clearer. It was in a good location. The ad jumped out at me. *Man! This will have more responses than the previous ad.*

That morning at church, I was walking around the outside of one of the buildings and approached Jody to say hello. He was talking with some woman I did not know. He saw me and said, "Hey, Mike, I almost didn't recognize you with your clothes on."

"Did you see Mike modeling his bod in the newspaper this morning," he asked the woman.

"No, but I am going home now to get my paper," she said.

We laughed and started talking about the weight I lost and how I did it.

My friend, Big O, called to put it in his normal acid voice, said. "You tightwad! How much did they pay you? It must have been a fortune for you to let them put them ugly pictures of you in the paper."

Martha was getting calls. She was not a happy camper. Her response was, "This was a sensitive subject."

Just recently she had to visit Dr. Uro. He saw the ad and mentioned it to her. He wanted to know how "the stud" was doing.

CHAPTER 26
CLOSING THOUGHTS

In an earlier chapter, I mentioned that the life expectancy of doing nothing about having prostate cancer was approximately ten years. Had I not had my prostate removed, that amount of time for me would have ended around 2011. It is now 2017.

My health is good. My life has been great, thanks to Martha, Michael, Molly, Miles, Annabelle, Walker, my dad, and my brothers and their families (plus friends and relatives). Being alerted that my life could end in ten years gave me a reason to extend that period. We all benefit by enjoying the moment. Nobody knows when our lives will be over.

How do we enhance quality of life? Living in good health requires our constant attention. We must keep a maintenance schedule for healthy living.

Just recently I had acid indigestion. I visited Dr. Intern. He recommended I stop caffeine: coffee, tea, and sodas. Stop eating spicy foods.

Jokingly, I asked, "If I do that, what's left for me to enjoy?"

"Don't know, but it is your decision."

He and I are the same age. We have had many conversations over the years. He doesn't beat around the bush.

Several years ago, we were talking about smoking. I do not smoke; it came up in a conversation. He said, "Smoking will kill people, maybe directly or indirectly. It kills people. I have seen too much of it in my profession. Secondhand smoke is just as bad."

What would I have missed? The birth of my three grandchildren? Being a part of watching them grow? Michael's and Molly's growth as parents and adults? Martha and I actively being involved?

Martha and I have always enjoyed being around people. Both of us gather socially with friends. Both of us have a set of people we get together with individually—laughing, eating, talking, and feeling comfortable with one another. It all deals with enjoying life.

My physical health is good for someone who is seventy years old. I try to work out, walk, and do what I can physically. Most important to me is stretching.

I work full-time. I enjoy the opportunity to be able to have a job and perform my duties at this age. Not that I am the ideal weight. From what I read, I am about fifteen pounds overweight. My only health restrictions result from the aging process, not from the prostate removal.

Mentally I have the signs of getting old just as we all do. They seem to come in spurts. Having a good memory recall was a huge plus for me. Now I am burdened when I cannot remember a person's name. I hate that I can't remember a ten-digit telephone number if someone tells it to me. Those things were easy for me years ago.

All over, there are articles about prostate cancer. Most are about the PSA test—the accuracy of it. Is it reliable in detecting prostate cancer? Should doctors even use it today?

I read a recent article concerning the reliability of the PSA test. As I stated earlier, several factors unrelated to prostate cancer can affect the results. There is a good possibility the results can vary from facility to facility analyzing the results.

I read another article about what it means if one has a biop-sy showing cancer cells in the prostate. Even if cancer cells are there, does it matter? The cells may be there for many years and not spread from the prostate. It's not so bad as long as the cancer does not leave the prostate.

It is your life. You need to be aware of what's taking place. All the diets recommended may have some validity. One of my rec-ommendations was to eat tomatoes to reduce the risk of prostate cancer. Heck, I have eaten more tomatoes than the number of to-matoes starring in the movie *Attack of the Killer Tomatoes*. It didn't help. They told me to eliminate fried food in my diet. I would hate to go through life not knowing what a hamburger tastes like—or even that foreign food, french fries.

Being able to write about my experience some fifteen years later is all the confirmation I need to know that Martha, my urolo-gist, and I made the right decisions. My hope for you is that you make the right decisions for your situation.

Remember, never give up.

ABOUT THE AUTHOR

MICHAEL HONEYCUTT SR. had prostate cancer. He has been cancer free for sixteen years.

He has been married to Martha Phillips Honeycutt for forty-six years. They currently live in Spartanburg, SC with their fickle feline, Speckles.

They have one son, Michael Honeycutt Jr. and his wife Molly, and three beautiful grandchildren.

He has a degree in Business Administration from Limestone College in Gaffney, SC.

He was a bombardier navigator flying in US Navy jets. He made cruises on board the USS Forrestal, USS Ranger and USS Saratoga. He is a Vietnam veteran and received several prestigious medals such as the Air Medal, first and second Strike/Flight Award and the Navy Commendation Medal with the Combat Distinguishing Device.

He is coping with PTSD (Post Traumatic Stress Disorder). With the help of the Veterans Administration and Martha, he is applying similar principles used in his battle with prostate cancer.